BASICS FOR EVALUATING MEDICAL RESEARCH STUDIES
A Simplified Approach
And Why Your Patients Need You To Know This

Delfini Group Evidence-based Practice Series
Short How-to Guide Book

By Sheri Ann Strite and Michael E. Stuart MD

"Best help with evidence-based medicine available."
Marty Gabica, MD, Chief Medical Officer, *Healthwise*

First Edition: 07/2013
Delfini Group Publishing: Delfini Group LLC
http://www.delfinigrouppublishing.com

ISBN-13: 978-1490926193 (CreateSpace-Assigned)
ISBN-10: 1490926194

Cover Design: Sheri Ann Strite
Cover Photo: Bat Shunatona MD

Table of Contents

Before You Begin Reading This Short Book

This book is about how to **evaluate the reliability and clinical usefulness** of clinical trials. When we refer to "medical science," "medical research," "reading a study" or other more general terms, understand that we are most frequently referring to **clinical trials for interventions using a superiority design** unless otherwise specified.

References are labeled as [author name, year if multiple entries by the primary author]. The citation can be looked up in the alphabetized reference list near the end. The PubMed Identification (PMID) numbers in the citations can be entered into PubMed's search box to obtain the full study citation and abstract.

We also provide you with access information to a **Reader Resource** web page at the end where you can find additional resources including a **glossary**. This will include a **1-page critical appraisal checklist** that you can use to remind yourself of essential critical appraisal considerations as you read studies. In addition, a wealth of freely available and helpful resources can also be found at our website: http://www.delfini.org.

Disclaimer

Use of this information implies agreement to our Notices at— http://www.delfini.org/index_Notices.htm.

In addition, your use implies agreement to the following. **We make no warranty, express or implied, or representation as to the accuracy, sufficiency or continued currency of the information contained herein.** The information contained in this book and any information or documents from the Delfini website may not be appropriate for use in all circumstances. Information may not be up-to-date, and it is up to the user to update the information. **Critical appraisal is inexact and a process of discovery**; therefore, not all potential issues may have been identified in a review, and different reviewers may reasonably come to different conclusions. Also, be aware that **there are exceptions to everything** presented here, and there is much judgment required in critical appraisal. We simplify and generalize for pattern learning of core concepts. However, be aware that frequently the most correct answer to any critical appraisal question is, "It depends..."

~~~

IMPORTANT INSIGHTS FROM THE AUTHORS & THE KEY TO THIS SHORT HOW-TO GUIDE

Saving Lives, One Sentence at a Time

What if we told you that we believe that the misreading by many doctors of two sentences in a published research study abstract may have contributed to an estimated 27,785 heart attacks and sudden cardiac deaths over a four year period of time [Consumer Affairs]?

What if we told you that we could have taught these doctors how to understand these two sentences in five minutes or less?

This book is based on our popular **tool-based, simplified approach to understanding medical literature** that we have used to train thousands. In the roughly two to four hours that we estimate that it will take you to read this book, you will understand many essential concepts about what makes a clinical trial and other medical research on therapeutic interventions reliable and clinically useful. If you apply these skills, you will be better equipped to care for your patients and provide them with an opportunity for true informed consent—which they rightfully deserve and which the nearly 28,000 patients that we mention above doubtfully received.

And some good news! You will not have to have deep statistical expertise to evaluate whether or not most interventional research studies are likely to be reliable and clinically useful. In this book, we will cover a few very simple statistics that are very easy to understand and crucially important to determine how likely patients are to experience an outcome. What you will discover is that the primary key to understanding the reliability of the study is largely about study design, methodology, execution and study performance outcomes such as whether or not blinding was successful.

Our Focus for This Short Book

Our primary focus for this book is on **evaluating the reliability and clinical usefulness** of efficacy results of superiority trials of therapeutic interventions. Our remarks should be assumed to be within this context, unless otherwise specified. We will briefly comment on safety, other kinds of health care interventions and a few other kinds of health care study designs as well.

Our focus is on the process steps and considerations for **evaluating a single trial**—which we refer to as a **primary study**, meaning the original study research.

Sometimes researchers perform a collective analysis of multiple studies together and report on their findings. Such a review is called a **secondary study** and ideally is undertaken in a formal way, which is called a "**systematic review**" (for example, a meta-analysis is a kind of secondary study). In this book, we do not give guidance on evaluating secondary studies. However, at the end we will give you tips on resources for evaluating secondary studies.

By **secondary sources** we mean medical information sources that utilize primary and secondary studies. These would include clinical guidelines and recommendations, health care economic studies, protocols, etc. These too should be critically appraised, and we also provide tips on resources for evaluating these information sources.

Quick Facts

- When it comes to medical science, we have **three essential questions**:

    1. Is it true?

    2. Is it useful?

    3. Is it usable?

- However, much of the medical literature relied upon for health care decision-making is too flawed to be reliable or is not reported sufficiently to know, or it is not clinically useful in ways that are likely to help patients.

- Much of the time, the chief problems with medical research reliability are due to bias. Bias in studies tends to favor the intervention. Bias has been documented to distort results up to a relative 50 percent or more for many individual biases. We will give you more evidence about this later.

- The majority of professional health care decision-makers lack skills in evaluating medical research for validity (meaning "closeness to truth") and clinical usefulness. These skills are referred to as critical appraisal or evidology skills.

- Most physicians rely on abstracts which are frequently inaccurate. One study found that 18 to 68 percent of abstracts in 6 top-tier medical journals contained information not verifiable in the body of the article [Pitkin]. One study concluded that there may be considerable bias in p-values reported in abstracts [Gotzsche]. While sometimes one can determine if a study is not reliable by reading the abstract, it cannot be determined that a study is valid by reviewing the abstract alone.

- Acquiring basic critical appraisal skills is easy and does not involve "heavy lifting" over statistics.

- Effective critical appraisal is a combination of understanding critical appraisal concepts and applying clinical knowledge and critical thinking to continually ask, "Could anything explain the reported study results other than truth?"—truth, meaning a cause and effect relationship between a therapeutic intervention of interest and a clinical outcome.

- The goal of this book is to provide you with these skills to help you accomplish our overarching medical science questions: **is it true** and **is it useful**. But first, a little more background.

Why Reading this Short Book is So Important & Can Help You

Physicians, patients, health care leaders—in fact, all of us—are making health care decisions every day. Good decisions require good information. Every day patients are harmed and resources are wasted because they make decisions they would not have made if they had been better informed.

The Health Care Information Problem: A Lot of Research and A Lot of Potentially Untrustable Research

We have a large problem with the quality of information we get from the published medical literature.

- In discussions concerning the state of scientific knowledge, the Institute of Medicine (IOM) concluded that it was plausible that only 4 percent of interventions used in health care have strong evidence to support them [Field].

- And yet, we have a lot of studies. The National Library of Medicine (NLM) is the world's largest library. Each week, more than 13,000 references are added to it.

- Professor John Ioannidis "...charges that as much as 90 percent of the published medical information that doctors rely on is flawed [Freedman]."

- It is our estimate, having evaluated thousands of studies, that approximately less than 10 percent of published randomized controlled trials (RCTs) in the health care literature are both valid and clinically useful or reported sufficiently to tell.

- One large review of 60,352 studies reported that only 7 percent passed criteria of high quality methods and clinical relevancy [McKibbon].

- Fewer than 5 percent passed a validity screening for a highly respected evidence-based journal [Glasziou].

In most instances, it is only by conducting critical appraisals of the medical literature for validity and usefulness that we can determine if an intervention is likely to be effective. Safety information is usually quite limited, and months or years may pass before we truly know about safety—if ever.

Patients Deserve Critically Appraised Information: Key Points

Critical appraisal is the best method known for assessing if a research study is likely to be reliable—and the purpose of reliable research is to help improve the ability to predict what will happen to a patient.

- Only after the evidence has been critically appraised for validity can we conclude that beneficial outcomes reported in clinical trials were not caused or distorted by bias or chance.

- Patients deserve to know the benefits and risks of interventions and the likelihood of experiencing various outcomes. Without critical appraisal of the evidence, this is not possible.

- Patient preferences are very likely to differ if patients are provided with information about the quality of the evidence and the amount of benefit and risk.

We Cannot Just Rely Upon the FDA

Reliance upon the Food and Drug Administration (FDA) is insufficient for medical decision-makers' sole source of information about the safety and efficacy of drugs and devices. The agency, for example, does not provide any information about comparative efficacy and safety or cost. Also, there are many instances in which reviewers may disagree that there is sufficient evidence of efficacy and safety.

Everyone Involved in Research Should Be Assumed to Be Biased

Generally, in this book when we use the term "bias" we are not speaking of bias in a sense of a person having a biased opinion or leaning toward a particular point of view. Generally, we use **bias to mean that something about the study is leading us away from truth**, other than a chance effect. This might be a distortion in results due to lack of blinding, for example.

However, we do wish to make a few comments about the potential of biased investigators. Some people believe that a study should be disregarded as being biased simply because it is funded by a manufacturer. We think that it's important to make note of such a fact, but to exclude studies simply on this basis would result in missing much valid and important information. It is also important to keep in mind that almost anyone conducting or participating in research may be biased even in the absence of support of a commercial entity. People who conduct or participate in research are frequently rooting for the intervention being investigated. Academic researchers may want fame, may be under pressure to publish or may be competing for tenure, etc.

Things to Keep in Mind as You Read This Book

In this book, we will present our approach to the evaluation of a clinical trial. Our primary focus in this book is on **therapeutic interventions using a superiority design**. There are other kinds of health care interventions: "screening," "diagnostic" and "preventive" are the other three. Many of our comments apply to these as well, although there are some special additional considerations for screening and diagnostic testing. We will provide you with resources to help you evaluate these other kinds of interventions as well.

Even though there is no "best way" to critically appraise a clinical trial, we would like each reader to come away with important concepts and tools to effectively "read" a clinical trial which is often used as shorthand for saying "critically appraising a study for validity and clinical usefulness." While there are different approaches to evaluating a clinical trial, good appraisers have in common a good understanding of bias, confounding and chance, knowing the potential for these study flaws to distort study results, and they share an understanding of what constitutes clinical usefulness.

Although we wrote this book primarily for practicing physicians, residents and students for whom critical appraisal information is relatively new, we have written this book with other health care professionals, residents and students in mind, along with their teachers. In fact, this book is intended for **anyone** with an interest in understanding how to evaluate medical research. Whether you are a student or resident; a clinician such as a physician, pharmacist or nurse practitioner, etc.; a clinical improvement specialist; a researcher; a committee member (e.g., Pharmacy and Therapeutics Committee, Medical Technology Assessment Committee or Quality Improvement team, etc.); a medical leader; a medical writer; a legal professional or even a patient with an interest in medical research, you will benefit from having an understanding of how study flaws can affect reported study results and, you will benefit from having a systematic approach to evaluating studies for flaws. You will be better equipped to evaluate efficacy and safety results and conclusions presented in clinical trials. You will make better health care decisions.

The Two Sentences

You are probably curious about the two mystery sentences in the story we opened with. The VIGOR (Vioxx GI Outcomes Research) study was a clinical trial comparing the upper gastrointestinal toxicity of the COX-2 inhibitor, rofecoxib (trade name Vioxx), versus naproxen, an over-the-counter anti-inflammatory drug used for arthritis and pain in the same family as aspirin and ibuprofen [Bombardier]. The study was published in November 2000 in the New England Journal of Medicine (NEJM)—one of the most respected medical journals in the world—and many would say "the" most respected journal.

In their study, the authors concluded their abstract by saying that Vioxx is "...associated with significantly fewer clinically important upper gastrointestinal events...," meaning fewer serious stomach ulcer problems, "...than treatment with naproxen."

After the study came out, in the hallways of Group Health Cooperative where he worked, Mike kept running into gastrointestinal specialists, or GI docs, who were very excited. "A 60 percent reduction in ulcer complications!" they enthused. Many others all over the world were also clearly impressed because worldwide sales for Vioxx in 2001 were $2.6 billion, up 18 percent from 2000, and the medicine claimed half of the new prescriptions in its class of medicines. For the first quarter of 2002, sales were $650 million, compared with $485 million in the first quarter of 2001 [Merck Newsroom].

However, the results got attention because of *how* the results were reported. They were reported in the study abstract as a "relative risk" of GI complications of 0.4, P=0.005. Right now, all you need to know about this is that a relative risk of 0.4 means that, in comparing Vioxx to naproxen, the relative risk of the ulcer complications if you took Vioxx was 40 percent of the risk you would have if you had taken naproxen. A simpler way to say this is that the risk with Vioxx was reduced by 60 percent. Thus, doctors started talking about a 60 percent reduced risk with Vioxx. (The P=0.005 is the "P-value," and it is telling us that this outcome is statistically significant, which suggests there is a low likelihood that these findings were due to a fluke accident).

A 60 percent reduction in risk sounds very impressive. However, there is a missing piece of information here. The question doctors needed to ask was, "Sixty percent of what?" Not asking this question is metaphorically akin to seeing a discount tag in a store that something is marked 60 percent off, but not asking 60 percent of what and blindly handing over your credit card. In the case of Vioxx, the answer would have been 60 percent of less than one percent! So what sounded to be a big and impressive difference was, in fact, incredibly small.

Here are the facts:

The number of people who might have benefited from avoiding a serious stomach problem—for example, a bleeding ulcer—if taking Vioxx instead of naproxen was estimated as only one person out of 125 people. Many of us might consider this too potentially small a clinical benefit especially when taking into account unknown safety issues and costs of new agents.

However in this instance, the published study did report some very concerning safety data. Yet, somehow many physicians managed to overlook the data on heart attack that were also reported *right there in the abstract.* Unfortunately (amazingly!), physicians didn't seem to notice that it was possible that Vioxx was actually causing heart attacks in one out of 103 people taking the agent. Ultimately, other studies also showed that more people were harmed than helped by the drug, and the harm was worse than the ulcer problems the drug was supposed to reduce. If you ask physicians which of the two harms they would prefer—would they rather have a serious ulcer problem or a serious blood clot, stroke or heart attack?—every physician we've ever asked immediately answers that he or she would rather have the ulcer problem.

But there is an even bigger point here. Most doctors and patients started using a drug without carefully assessing the reliability of the information and accepted the reported benefits which were presented in a way that misled almost everyone. Plus they accepted the way the safety data were presented which suggested that naproxen conferred benefit, rather than what was really true: that Vioxx caused harm.

Our mission is to help you and others avoid a similar tragedy and also to help you better help patients and help yourself and your loved ones. Learning this information can be empowering. Our hope is that we will provide you with knowledge and skills that will serve you the rest of your life—and serve you personally when you or your loved ones are in the role of a patient.

~~~

The Goal of Clinical Trials

The goal of clinical trials for therapeutic interventions is to determine whether or not outcomes of interest are due to the intervention or due to some other factor. A key question we want to answer before seriously considering the study results of a clinical trial is whether the association between the intervention and the outcome is due to cause and effect or is due to bias or chance.

So this is our overarching question that guides our entire reading of a study:

Can anything explain the study results other than truth? In other words, what caused the outcome? And so ultimately, a primary goal of medical research is to determine causality.

Once we have critically appraised the trial in a systematic way and determined that the study is valid, we then evaluate the results for clinical usefulness by evaluating both benefits and harms. Patients benefit from effective therapeutic interventions when benefits outweigh harms, but we cannot know if an intervention is likely to be effective without critically appraising the studies reporting the results.

"Likely to be effective" is a key concept in evaluating the usefulness of clinical trials. Medications don't always work the same for everyone. And so we look to medical science to help answer who is likely to benefit and who is likely to experience a harm. We look at the number of events that occurred in a study to calculate how many people benefited or were harmed out of all of those treated and compare those numbers between study arms. Study arms may be more than two, but to simplify, we will generally stick to two groups in most examples. **So this is an overarching question that guides our assessment of**

results from a *valid* study:

What is the probability of benefit or harm? "External validity" is the term used when asking this question "for my patient" or "my population?"

Again, **safety information is usually quite limited**, and months or years may pass before we know about safety—if ever. So patients should generally always be advised that this can be an area of uncertainty.

But before we dive into the process we use to critically appraise clinical trials, we want to step back and consider the difference between experiments and observations and give you a few quick tips.

~~~

Study Design

The first step in assessing the validity of a study is to match the study design to the clinical question. Because our focus is on medical interventions, we are not going to review here appropriate study designs for other kinds of clinical questions. And unless you are planning to be a researcher, **we have good news**. Most epidemiology textbooks cover details of various study types—e.g., case-control, cohort studies, etc. Most health care professionals do not need to understand all these research study variations to understand how to evaluate the science about whether an intervention is likely to work or not or whether we have too little information to tell. Generally, all that is needed is to be able to **distinguish between observations and experiments**.

Observations and Experiments

At its most basic level, study designs are either observational or they are experiments.

Observations

In observations, you observe what happens naturally. Observations can be useful to answer certain questions, but they are highly prone to bias and can almost never be relied upon to answer questions about cause and effect. With observational studies, there is a lack of equality in many "prognostic factors" between studied groups. This lack of equality starts with how similar the groups are or are not to each other at the outset of their being observed, and this is a problem that cannot be sufficiently addressed through statistical adjusting because, at the very least, many differences are unknown. And this lack of equality between groups in observational studies may extend beyond the make-up of the groups studied to various areas as differences in care such as in co-interventions or care experiences, measurement methods, length of time followed and more.

Observational studies have their uses. They are important for hypothesis-generating, and they can tell us many helpful things about patient care such as prognosis and natural history of a disease. They can be suggestive of safety issues. They can inform us about important issues such as adherence and clinical questions about current practice, etc. But with rare exception (i.e., "all-or-none" results*), they cannot be trusted to answer questions of cause and effect.

Experiments

With very rare exception,* an experiment is the only way to establish cause and effect, and for important reasons, valid randomized controlled trials (the RCT being the highest quality type of experimental design) are the very best way to determine if a therapeutic intervention is effective.

So this is the first of our Quick Tips:

Did the patient or his or her physician *choose* the patient's treatment? If yes, this is an observational study, and with the very rare occasion of all-or-none results*, you can ignore the study if you are seeking information about efficacy.

"Efficacy" simply refers to "research study results of benefit to study patients" (contrasted with what benefits to patients may be expected in real world application, which is termed, "effectiveness").

*"All-or-none results" is the term that is used when highly dramatic differences in outcomes between groups are observed. For example, before the intervention, everyone died; after application of the intervention, almost no one died. When all-or-none results occur in observational studies, they are generally considered reliable. But only well-done experiments with good study performance outcomes are considered truly reliable to establish cause and effect.

We will also give you another **Quick Tip**:

Unless we are doing an extensive safety review, **when we are evaluating the medical literature to learn about the efficacy or the safety of an intervention, we almost never spend any time reviewing observational studies.** When using PubMed, which is the user interface to the United States National Library of Medicine (NLM), we usually limit our medical literature searches to "*clinical trials.*" While there are other kinds of experiments, studies are at great risk of producing misleading results if the groups to be compared are not equivalent.

When an experiment is done correctly with successful study performance outcomes—and here comes **the clinical trial at its essence** that you will want to make sure that you understand—we repeat: it is the only truly reliable way to establish cause and effect.

The Successful Clinical Trial Boiled Down

The scientific method requires, in most instances, that there are **at least two concurrent groups** for study in clinical trials. At the most basic level, one intervention is pitted against another intervention in an experimental study, which includes placebo or "to usual care," and the outcomes in the groups are compared.

- To determine cause and effect, you need to compare one thing to something else and—this is most important—you need to **isolate those two things to make an effective comparison—meaning everything else in your experiment must be completely the same for those factors (e.g., drug versus placebo) to be isolated.**

- To do so, you need a group of people that makes sense to study.

- To keep everything the same, you want to divide your study participants into comparison groups in a way that results in each of the **groups being as similar as possible.** (This will be one of four key benefits of using a randomized approach, or "minimization" which we will discuss later.) You want to do this because you do not want a difference between the groups— instead of what you are studying—to be a cause of the results or to distort them in some way.

- You want to **eliminate any choice of treatment** because people choose treatments for different reasons, and a reason for choosing a treatment may result in other kinds of choices that will make the comparison groups different. So you need a way to assign treatments which takes choice out of the equation. (This is the second of four key benefits of randomization.)

- You want to **treat your groups exactly the same** except for what you are studying—meaning the intervention of interest and what it is being compared to—so that some other difference between the groups isn't the cause or a distorter of the results.

- You want to **successfully measure** the resulting outcomes of interest, and you want those **outcomes to be of importance** to patients (e.g., reduced mortality, relief from pain, etc.)—and you want them to be **true** (e.g., **not distorted by bias, not a result of chance** and **not be a false negative because your groups were too small to experience outcomes of interest**).

- And here comes another important key that will become fundamental to your understanding the operation of various study biases—**clinical trials are about comparing the resulting differences between the groups**. When we talk about "research results," we are talking about the "difference in outcomes between the groups." And you want those differences to be of **sufficient size to matter**—which is context-dependent and a matter of judgment.

That's it! That's a quality clinical trial in a nutshell. How you achieve this has a lot of other pieces to it—such as how blinding can be so important in helping to ensure that the groups are treated the same.

Problems with Observational Research

In observations, investigators simply gather information about what transpires, resulting from patients and their doctors (or other health care professionals) choosing a therapy. And choice can carry with it many differences between groups as to why they made a choice which can dramatically affect—and often explain—study results. Experiments remove the element of choice, thereby reducing the risk of biases that arise because of different choices made by people with different needs, wants, prognoses, lifestyles, cultures, limitations, abilities, values, preferences, etc. which we refer to as "patient requirements."

A good example of being misled about cause and effect associations is the hormone replacement therapy (HRT) saga. Several decades ago, doctors observed and published research about their experiences using hormone replacement therapy (e.g., estrogen preparations) for the treatment of women who had experienced myocardial infarctions (MIs). Women who had experienced an MI were treated with HRT because numerous observational studies reported that women who took HRT had lower rates of second MIs—in other words, HRT was associated with having fewer additional MIs when compared to women not treated with HRT. Many physicians told women that they believed that there were beneficial effects of HRT in preventing second MIs because they relied on what are now known to be low quality studies (i.e., observations).

Observational studies are likely to report misleading results—in fact, the chance of an observational study for therapy being correct may be as low as 20 percent [Ioannidis 05]. In this case, the low quality observational studies reported lower rates of MI in women who chose to take HRT, *which was a true finding*, but the doctors concluded that the lower rate of heart attacks was *due to taking HRT*. In fact, what probably happened was that the women who chose to take HRT were different from the women who did not choose to take HRT. The women taking HRT may have been especially interested in their health, which was the reason for their taking the drug, and also they most likely took better care of themselves (e.g., exercised, made better dietary choices, etc.), and that was the likely explanation for the lower rate of heart attacks in these women. Finally, valid RCTs showed that women with documented coronary artery disease did not benefit from HRT, and there were increased rates of harms such as breast cancer, blood clots and stroke. After these studies were published, many doctors stopped telling women who had suffered MIs that HRT had been shown in medical studies to prevent future MIs [Ioannidis 01].

The HRT saga illustrates the big problem of selection bias and how poor quality evidence can mislead us. Therefore, an initial step in critical appraisal of therapeutic interventions is determining if the study is an observational study or an experiment. Once this has been accomplished, you can move on to evaluating whether the study is likely to be useful or not—*if true!*—and we will get to "if true" after a few more **Quick Tips**. There is no point in spending time evaluating a research study if it isn't going to be useful. In our workshops, we admonish new learners, "Don't even *look at the results* until you know the study is likely to be true." And we say this because people are at risk of biasing themselves into believing the results just by reading them. But because we want to save everyone time, we then say, "Okay, you can *peek* at them, but only to quickly establish whether it is worth your time to critically appraise the study. And then you have to forget the reported results until you know that the study is valid."

~~~

Quick Tips for Initially Assessing Possible Usefulness of a Clinical Trial

If the Results are Reliable, Are They Useful?

Will these results change practice? Will patients benefit?

1. Are the reported **results big enough to benefit patients in clinically meaningful ways?** An **outcome**—also referred to as an "endpoint"—is what we are interested in studying. Typically these are **events** that patients experience such as pain or mortality, and studies may focus on reduction in events such as "reduction in mortality" or they may focus on improvements such as in "improved quality of life." Another synonym to outcome or endpoint is "outcome measure," which is sometimes shorted to "measure," and frequently, we will refer to "events." Clinical trials are about comparing the difference in the number of experienced events between the study groups—and this is where "big enough" comes in. (As to "big enough," keep in mind the Vioxx saga and how results that seemed large were actually very small.) Later in the book, we will give you tips to answer this question including instructions on how to use confidence intervals which can be informative.

Generally an investigator chooses a "primary outcome" of interest to study—or possibly two—and a series of other areas of interest called "secondary outcomes." Research that benefits patients in clinically meaningful ways addresses 5 key areas—and these are important to always keep in mind: 1) **morbidity**; 2) **mortality**; 3) **symptom relief**; 4) mental, physical and emotional **functioning**; and, 5) health-related **quality of life.**

About Intermediate Markers: If an endpoint does not fall into one of these 5 topic areas, then it is called an intermediate outcome marker, some synonyms for which include "intermediate markers," "proxy markers," "surrogate markers" and "surrogate endpoints." An intermediate marker represents an outcome that is not directly experienced by people—blood pressure, lab or imaging tests, for example. Intermediate markers are outcome measures that are "assumed" to represent clinical outcomes—meaning these outcomes that we listed above that matter to patients. But they may or may not truly predict a clinically useful outcome. As an example, "blood pressure" is often used as a surrogate endpoint in studies of stroke when the clinically significant outcome we are actually hoping to achieve is "reduction in stroke," which falls into the clinically significant categories of morbidity and mortality that we reviewed earlier. Effective critical appraisal requires a direct causal chain of proof of meaningful clinical benefit to accept the value of an intermediate marker.

The encainide/flecainide [Echt] example is instructive not only about the risk of assuming the relatedness of an intermediate marker to a clinical outcome, but also about what can happen when treatments become established through simple observations or through pathophysiological reasoning instead of through high quality science. In the mid-1980s, it was observed that patients who experienced premature ventricular contractions—or PVCs—after acute myocardial infarction had a higher risk of mortality than patients who did not experience PVCs. Because encainide and flecainide were agents that could suppress PVCs, their use became common in medical practice—without valid science supporting their use. By 1990, roughly 50 percent of all US cardiologists were estimated to be using these agents [Morganroth]. This stopped when a randomized controlled trial showed that patients on these agents were more likely to die than those who took placebo. Approximately 8.3 percent of patients with PVCs who took these medications would be likely to die or experience a cardiac death over 10 months as compared to about 3.5 percent of patients taking placebo. We estimate that possibly roughly 63,000 preventable deaths occurred due to use of these agents. Compare that to the Vietnam War in which it is estimated that 58,000 US lives were lost [Digital History].

Sometimes researchers combine outcomes together to create one single measure such as "all-cause mortality." When individual endpoints are grouped together to create a single measure, they are called composite outcomes or composite endpoints. For example, an outcome of "major cardiovascular events" might consist of the individual measures of cardiovascular death plus nonfatal myocardial infarction plus stroke. An important critical appraisal consideration is whether the composite measure is a meaningful one and if it is a fair one.

There are many considerations in evaluating a composite endpoint, but the relatedness of the individual outcomes is an important issue when assessing whether it is a meaningful one. "Fairness" too has a number of considerations. A classic one is that whatever is the most frequent event is going to be the driver of the outcome. Imagine a composite endpoint called "major stroke events" in which "stroke" is combined with "hospitalization for any reason." A physician researcher could impact the number of outcomes by choosing to hospitalize a study patient, thereby increasing "major stroke events."

2. Will these results be **applicable to my patients**? A key consideration is what is referred to as "**external validity**" which means "how likely are the study results to be true in my circumstances?" For example, do you consider your patients similar enough to the patients studied that you believe that the results will apply to your patients? To assess this you want to look at the inclusion and exclusion criteria and, importantly, the baseline characteristics of the patients studied. You may want to take a look at other contextual issues too such as the setting for care and likelihood of successful execution of the treatment or factors which may affect adherence.

A useful framework for an external validity assessment, among other things, is PICOTS which stands for patient, intervention, comparator, outcome, timing and setting [Atkins 08].

3. Is the **comparison fair?**

4. Were research questions, outcomes for study and analysis groups **determined in advance** or *a priori*? If not, there is a high risk that the reported results are due to chance.

5. Was the clinical trial **halted early** for efficacy, and are there fewer than 500 events? If yes, there may be a high risk that the reported results are due to chance.

6. Do you agree with **how the researchers defined outcomes** such as success/failure, improvement/no improvement, etc.?

7. And always be mindful that, if this study is for a new agent, **safety is likely to be unknown**.

If you are satisfied with the answers to these questions, you can now move to a closer assessment of the study methods, execution and study performance outcomes to gauge the likelihood of study reliability and relevance. This is an assessment of "internal validity" which means "how likely are the study results to be true in the context of the research study?"

We summarize our quick tips in a 1-pager that you can download from our **Reader Resource** web page.

~~~

Bias, Confounding and Chance

We will now review some key concepts related to critical appraisal. First, there are **4 explanations for the association**—or the relationship—between the study interventions and the study results. They can be explained by—

- **Bias**: something that "systematically" leads away from truth ("systematically" simply meaning not random chance);

- **Confounding**: a special form of bias in which we think something has caused an outcome, but it is something else— hence we are "confounded" or confused by the confounder*;

- **Chance**: random accident; or,

- **Cause and effect**: truth.

*A classic example of confounding is in research reporting that taking vitamins reduces the risk of coronary heart disease when, in fact, people who take vitamins are more likely to do other things which reduce this risk. So in this instance, supplementary vitamin intake is the confounder, and healthy lifestyle is the actual cause.

A major goal of critical appraisal is to uncover bias, confounding and chance effects that may distort the reported study results. If we can rule out these potential explanations for the reported study results, then we can conclude that the results are likely to be because of causality—meaning that the results are due to the intervention being studied. For this reason, critical appraisal largely focuses on study problems, not on positive aspects of studies.

Also, sometimes good study design cannot be followed and study performance outcomes may fail. It would be unethical to randomize patients to smoke cigarettes or not, for example, and it is sometimes impossible to blind a treatment. A critical appraisal cannot "forgive" these impossibilities in bias assessment because reality does not make an "allowance" for difficulty, and it is not the efforts of the researchers that are being evaluated, but how confident we are in the study findings.

Many people are under the impression that misapplied statistics are the biggest problem resulting in unreliable research. But that is not true, and many biostatisticians agree that the biggest problems in research generally arise because of bias. So let's take a general look at bias a little more closely.

More on Bias

Remember that **bias is anything that systematically leads away from truth**. (Because confounding is a special form of bias, from here on we will frequently just refer to bias.) And also remember that to determine cause and effect, we need groups to compare that are identical except for the one thing we are studying. We then look at results to see if the groups differed.

> **Quick Tip**: **Any difference between groups other than what is being studied is automatically a bias** because that difference could explain or distort study results.

Anything else (other than chance) which can distort the results is a bias. So another example would be faulty measuring methods applied equally to both groups. Bias can distort study efficacy results by overestimating or underestimating benefits; however, research has shown again and again that bias tends to favor the intervention. Some biases are considered lethal threats and others are considered minor threats. As the Cochrane Handbook points out, it is not possible to accurately predict how much over- or underestimation of the true intervention effect is caused by a particular flaw in a particular trial [Higgins]. However, researchers who study the effects of various biases on results by comparing study results from trials with specific biases compared to similar studies without the biases have frequently been able to isolate relative percentages of distortion in the studies they have reviewed. We present these estimated ranges simply to illustrate that bias can have a meaningful impact on study results. These researchers have found distortion of results by less than a relative 5 percent to more than 50 percent [Chalmers 83, Moher 98, Kjaergard 01, van Tulder 09, Lachin 00, Savovic 12].

A common result of not critically appraising studies before considering study results is that the evidence gets "upgraded," meaning that lower quality studies are judged to be at lower risk of bias than they really are [Kjaergard 01, Reichenbach]—or labeled as if they are of higher quality. This, in turn, frequently results in accepting results suggesting more benefit than actually exists or—worse—accepting study results reporting benefit when no benefit exists [Reichenbach].

If a clinical trial is free from bias and the results are not due to chance, the study is said to be "internally valid," which is frequently referred to as study quality or the methodological quality of a study. We will now examine the 4 key steps in assessing bias in a clinical trial which roughly correspond to the flow of a trial, and we will present some data that will give you some idea of the range of distortion that has been found to occur with study flaws. We concentrate on RCTs because a clinical trial that does not utilize randomization (or minimization) to allocate subjects to their study groups is already at significant risk of bias.

An important point to keep in mind in reviewing the steps, is that, in reading a trial, you may discover something else that you think may explain or distort results. Anything that leads away from truth in a study (other than chance) is a bias whether you see it on a list of considerations or not.

~~~

The 4 Key Steps for Assessing Bias in a Clinical Trial

There are four stages of a clinical trial and some key questions associated with evaluating bias in each of those stages.

1. **Subject Selection & Treatment Assignment**

    Important considerations include who was studied, how were they selected for study, are there enough people, how were they assigned to their study groups, and are the groups balanced.

2. **Study Performance: Intervention & Context**

    What is being studied, and what is it being compared to? What else happened to study subjects in the course of the study?

3. **Data Collection & Loss of Data**

    What information was collected, and how was it collected? What data are missing, and do missing data meaningfully distort the study results?

4. **Results & Assessing The Differences In The Outcomes Of The Study Groups**

    How is the difference in outcomes between the groups evaluated? What are those differences and how are they expressed?

And after you evaluate a study for bias, you then assess the likelihood of chance. If the study is valid and the risk of chance is low, then you want to evaluate meaningful clinical benefit and the potential for harm.

Before we get started in detailing how to apply these questions, we're going to first show you an example of a critical appraisal. The case below is a fictional one. We present first the study abstract from a hypothetical journal, followed by our critical appraisal in which we list the hypothetical threats to validity in this made-up study.

Important: In looking at this example, keep in mind that we have only presented an abstract here. Abstracts can sometimes be useful by themselves to determine if a study is worth evaluating. However, abstracts are insufficient for determining that a study is valid. In this case, we are not showing you the "full published study." This example is to show you what a critical appraisal may look like.

DELFINI CRITICAL APPRAISAL CASE STUDY

HYPOTHETICAL CASE STUDY

MYOCEPTIMAB PREVENTS CARDIOVASCULAR MORBIDITY

Critical Appraisers & Date: Sheri A. Strite & Michael E. Stuart MD, Delfini Group; April Fool's Day, Any Year

PUBLISHED ABSTRACT

Background

Elevated myoreactive protein has been demonstrated to be associated with increased risk of myocardial infarction (MI). Myoceptimab is an inhibitor of myoreactive protein and has been shown to reduce myoreactive protein levels.

Methods

We conducted a randomized, double-blind trial in the Beaverton University Heart Care Center to assess the efficacy and safety in patients ages 55 and older who were at increased risk for cardiovascular events and had elevated myoreactive protein levels above 4 mg/L on two separate occasions. Patients were randomly assigned to receive 60 mg of myoceptimab (29 patients) or placebo (35 patients) daily for 6 months.

The study outcome was cardiovascular morbidity as defined by mean reduction of elevated levels of myoreactive protein, onset of new angina, admission to the hospital for any cardiovascular-related condition, myocardial infarction, stroke, claudication, heart failure or cardiovascular death.

Results

At 6 months, active treatment resulted in significantly reduced mean levels of myoreactive protein by 37%, reduced cardiovascular morbidity (n = 19 [65.5%] vs. n = 7 [20%]; P = 0.0003), and significantly more patients had a >50% increase in quality of life. There were no reported differences in safety outcomes.

Conclusions

Treatment with myoceptimab reduced cardiovascular morbidity and was associated with significant beneficial effects on quality of life. Myoceptimab offers a safe and effective therapeutic option for patients who are at increased risk for cardiovascular events.

DELFINI CRITICAL APPRAISAL

- Study size: small
- Primary endpoint: questionable composite
- Randomization: not truly randomized; patients assigned to groups by study consent date
- Concealment of allocation: no details
- Baseline characteristics: slightly higher rate of angina in the placebo group
- Blinding: insufficient details and no indication of blind assessment
- Intergroup differences: participating cardiologists were not restricted in patient management so as to replicate real-world conditions; no details of co-interventions reported between groups
- Attrition: less than 1 percent
- Safety, including long term harms, is uncertain
- Results assessment: questionable clinical significance, selective reporting and *post-hoc* results
- Critical appraisal conclusion: uncertain validity

Step 1. Subject Selection & Treatment Assignment— Evaluating a Clinical Trial for Selection Bias

5 Essential Questions for Assessing Selection Bias:

1. Who was studied?

2. How were they selected for study?

3. Are there enough people?

4. How were they assigned to their study groups?

5. Are the groups balanced?

1. Who Was Studied

Review the inclusion criteria and exclusion criteria. This is akin to the invitation list to the party. Use clinical knowledge and critical thinking to reason through whether these seem to be the right people for study. For example, a study that includes people who previously failed the comparator would stack the deck in favor of the intervention under study (and yes, we have seen this happen). We would consider this a lethal threat to validity and be likely to stop reading right there.

Also consider whether there is a likelihood of misdiagnosis. This might require taking an additional step of critically appraising a study of a diagnostic test. (Evaluating diagnostic tests is beyond the scope of this book, but we will provide a few core questions that are essential for critically appraising studies of diagnostic tests.)

Review the baseline characteristics. This is akin to who actually showed up at the party. Baseline characteristics should be reported for each group, keeping in mind that you should see reported key prognostic variables such as demographic and key disease characteristics (examples: age, sex, comorbidities, etc.). Keep in mind that investigators have a certain amount of control over which patient characteristics to measure and report. If something you think important is missing, that could be a red flag. Also, keep in mind that investigators can only measure what is measurable and report on what they measured. How likely is it that they were able to do an accurate measurement, assessment or diagnosis, for example? Unreported, unmeasured and unmeasurable characteristics cannot be evaluated.

2. How were they selected for study?

Often you won't find this information directly reported. But if it is disclosed, it is worth looking at. A study comparing the benefits of "exercise" compared to "no exercise" is unlikely to have adherent participants in the "no exercise group" if study subjects are recruited from the local gym.

3. Are there enough people?

Another important issue is the size of the study. A study with fewer than 100 participants is generally considered small, and small studies can be more prone to chance results. A small study can be valid and likely to be true—but generally should be viewed with caution.

Small studies can also be too small to find important outcomes—this is especially true when it comes to safety which we will discuss later when we discuss confidence intervals and show you some clues that might answer this question.

Because of concerns that a study might be too small to find a beneficial effect, researchers perform power calculations in an attempt to determine the minimum number of people they estimate that they need to enroll in a study. The **good news** is that, unless you are a researcher, you do not need to understand how power calculations are performed, and unless you are a researcher who is planning to further study this topic, you do not need to evaluate their calculation. Soon we will share with you the one easy thing you do need to know about "power," but it won't involve the power calculation.

4. How were they assigned to their study groups?

There are two key considerations: the allocation of patients to their study groups and hiding the allocation to those groups.

Allocation to Study Group

Investigators attempt to establish groups which have similar known and unknown characteristics (prognostic variables) to ensure that the reported effects of the intervention under study are not due to important baseline differences in prognostic variables between groups. Therefore, a critically important issue is whether subjects were assigned to their groups in ways that make balance between the groups likely.

Randomization is the best method we have to attempt to create equal groups at the start of a study. Randomization is important for four crucial reasons, some of which we have discussed: 1) randomization helps establish cause and effect because it is likely to evenly distribute known and unknown confounders between groups; 2) it eliminates confounding that can result from patient or provider choice of the intervention; and, 3) it creates an unpredictable method for assignment to a group which helps prevent someone manipulating the assignment of an intervention to a study subject (and yes, this does happen—and more frequently than you would suspect). A by-product of this—and the fourth key benefit—is that unpredictable group assignment is necessary for effective blinding. Methods such as alternation, date of birth or admission to the hospital are regarded as inadequate because of the possibility of "directing" certain patients into preferred groups [Van Tulder, Higgins]. And should this happen, the study may no longer be "blindable" regardless of specific blinding steps such as identical study capsules.

If subjects are not assigned to their study groups through randomization,* then the experiment can be highly prone to bias because the groups of subjects are likely to be different from each other, and those differences could affect or explain the study results.

Inadequate generation of the randomization sequence has been found to distort study results as high as a relative 75 percent.

(Keep in mind that these numbers are what we have found reported by various researchers. The effect of a distortion of results by bias could be much less, depending upon the specific study circumstance, or a discovered bias might not even cause a distortion in results—but it also could be that a bias causes a higher distortion. So we present these numbers mainly just to make you aware that bias can cause problems with results.)

It is possible that a non-random process called "minimization" may also evenly distribute prognostic variables, but we have restricted our discussion to randomization for the purposes of this book. With the single exception of "randomization," everything we say about RCTs applies to trials using minimization methods for allocating subjects to their study group.

Important Point: In order to effectively critically appraise a study, the appraiser **needs to evaluate specific details** of how various study procedures were conducted. **It is not sufficient for an article to simply state that a study was randomized.** Critical appraisers need more information such as, "Randomization was achieved through a computer-generated random number table to allocate study subjects to the study drug or to placebo." When key study details are not reported, the uncertainty about what was done should be recorded as a potential problem, such as "threat to validity" or as "uncertain risk of bias," as examples. There exists compelling evidence that when there is uncertainty about risk of bias, frequently bias is, in fact, present and distorting results [Hartling].

Tip: Sometimes the trial protocol or supplementary study information can fill in gaps. However, be aware that just because something is reported in a protocol, does not mean that the protocol has been followed. At times, we also will write the authors. Our advice is to be extremely clear about what you are asking and save all your questions for one correspondence. Frequently, you will not get a reply back, but if you do, you want to maximize your chances for getting the information you need.

Concealment of Allocation to Study Group

Another key selection bias is whether or not people can discover an upcoming assignment to a study group before a subject has actually been assigned. This is important because someone enrolling patients or assigning them to the study groups may manipulate the assignment in order to direct patients to a study arm they favor, such as directing higher risk patients to more conservative interventions or directing sicker patients to specific—and frequently newer—treatments because of a hope that they might be better. This kind of bias is referred to as "confounding by indication," which we will discuss in greater detail later.

The term for hiding the allocation to groups is "concealment of allocation," which is a type of blinding—but note that conventionally the term "blinding" is reserved for masking the study intervention after allocating patients to their groups. Inadequately concealed studies have been found to distort results as much as a relative 73 percent. Concealment is successful if no one is able to determine to which group the next subject will be allocated.

Methods to conceal allocation include the use of centralized call centers, computerized interactive voice response systems and identical locked containers to hide the allocation code, as examples. Sometimes you will see that opaque envelopes are used; however, envelopes can be easily manipulated—so we would look for additional protections before accepting this method.

5. Are the groups balanced?

Comparing baseline characteristics can be a clue as to whether randomization resulted in balanced groups or not. But it is only a clue and cannot be relied upon to ascertain adequacy of randomization.

Sometimes investigators indicate which characteristics have statistically significant differences between groups. Statistical significance, which we will discuss in greater detail later, pertains to a likelihood of chance effects. We do not find this very helpful when evaluating the table of baseline characteristics because, if an effective randomization process was used, *de facto* the differences are due to chance. We find it more helpful to apply clinical thinking to review the numbers reported in the table and gestalt a possible effect on results. But this is frequently unreliable at best, unless there are large differences. We've seen an instance where a combination of slight differences made a meaningful difference in study results.

List 1. Relative Distortion of Study Results in Clinical Trials Associated with Selection Bias (Researchers and PMID Numbers)

List 1 provides a range of reported distortions resulting from inadequate generation of the randomization sequence and other major selection biases, but it should be emphasized that the amount of distortion in clinical trials is likely to vary depending upon the condition being studied, the comparison intervention, the frequency of occurrence of the endpoint and other factors. Following our evaluation, we frequently rate the risk of bias for generation of the randomization sequence as high, low or uncertain as outlined in the Cochrane Handbook [Higgins]. We also frequently rate the other 3 areas of a clinical trial using this rating scheme.

Inadequate Generation of Sequence—estimated range unclear* to 75%

Juni 01 PMID: 11440947
Kjaergard 01PMID: 11730399
Savovic 12 PMID: 22945832
van Tulder 09 PMID: 19770609

Savovic 2012: PMID 22945832 found in a study of 1,973 trials up to 26% distortion if the endpoint was subjective or mixed, 18% overall, but unclear distortion if the endpoint was mortality or other objective endpoint.

Inadequate Concealment of Allocation of the Randomization Sequence—estimated range unclear * to 73%

Chalmers 83 PMID: 6633598
Juni 01 PMID: 11440947
Kjaergard 01 PMID: 11730399
Moher 98 PMID: 9746022
Savovic 12 PMID: 22945832
Schulz 95 PMID: 7823387

Savovic 12 PMID 22945832 found in a study of 1,973 trials up to 15% distortion if the endpoint was subjective or mixed, 13% overall, but unclear distortion if the endpoint was mortality or other objective endpoint.

~~~

Step 2. Study Performance: The Intervention and Context—Evaluating a Clinical Trial for Performance Bias

2 Essential Questions for Assessing Performance Bias

1. What is being studied and what is it being compared to?

2. What else happened to study subjects in the course of the study?

1. What is being studied and what is it being compared to?

In the performance stage, patients receive either the intervention being studied or the comparison experience. This is frequently a placebo, a sham procedure, another intervention or, at times, assignment to a "waiting list" or to receive usual care. The intervention that is the subject of interest in the study is referred to as the "intervention group" or the "study group" even if it is being compared to another active intervention.

What is being studied?

The "what is being studied" question is not just about what intervention is being studied—it is also about the outcomes the researcher has decided he or she wishes to evaluate. If you followed our early suggestions in **Quick Tips for Initially Assessing Possible Usefulness of a Clinical Trial: If the Results are Reliable, Are They Useful?**, you will already have attended to the important considerations concerning this question. You will have given thought to whether this is an intervention that you might use in practice. You will have paid attention to the outcomes of interest. You will have assessed whether the researcher has chosen to study clinically meaningful outcomes.

> **Important Point & Quick Tip**: A reminder that clinical outcomes are things that a patient can experience, and these are: 1) morbidity; 2) mortality; 3) symptom relief; 4) functioning; and, 5) quality of life. We think that these are important enough that they should be committed to memory because that will speed up your ability to quickly determine whether a study is worth paying attention to. A quick way to begin to lock this into memory is to start with the M&Ms, as they say (morbidity, mortality...)

If the researcher has chosen to study something other, then you will have determined, or will be alert for reasonable proof through valid evidence, that the intermediate outcome marker utilized has a proven direct causal chain to a meaningful clinical outcome.

You will have already evaluated the reasonableness of any composite outcomes.

What is it being compared to?

One key question: is the comparator fair? If a comparison medication is suboptimal, there is a high likelihood that the study drug will achieve better outcomes.

If the study is a head-to-head trial—such as when two active agents are compared to each other—is there a placebo arm and, if not, are there other valid data comparing the agents against placebo—or even against no treatment? This is important because effects may be masked without such a comparison. Remember the problems with the VIGOR trial [Bombardier]. Rofecoxib was compared to naproxen and there was no placebo arm. The study authors claimed that, "[Our] results are consistent with the theory that naproxen has a coronary protective effect and highlight the fact that rofecoxib does not provide this type of protection owing to its selective inhibition of cyclooxygenase-2 at its therapeutic doses and at higher doses."

Which led to this statement in the abstract: "The incidence of myocardial infarction was lower among patients in the naproxen group than among those in the rofecoxib group..." Truuuuuuuuue. But it was also true that the incidence of myocardial infarction was higher among patients in the rofecoxib group than among those in the naproxen group. Their theory was wrong, in fact. By comparing two active agents, uncertainty in safety was created because there was no placebo comparison which would have clearly revealed that the MIs were due to rofecoxib.

Most readers of this study did not possess critical appraisal skills and did not apply critical thinking to say, "Wait a minute! None of this was proved, and there is a potentially huge safety issue here!" Instead, lack of awareness of the large volume of problematic studies, lack of knowledge of how to evaluate studies and trust in the peer-reviewed journal process—*this was published in the New England Journal of Medicine, after all*—led to enormous problems for patients and many fatalities before the drug was pulled from the market.

2. What else happened to study subjects in the course of the study?

There are many other areas to examine when looking for performance bias. Here are some items that are typically considered in this stage: successful application of the intervention, medication adherence, patients getting the wrong treatment (contamination or migration) and other protocol violations, use of co-interventions, other care experiences, impacts of time and change, length of duration of treatment and length of study follow-up. For example, might the time period of the study affect study results (e.g., studying an allergy medication, but not during allergy season)? Is the duration of follow-up sufficient for patients to experience the outcome under study?

In addition to groups being balanced, everything else must be identical except for the intervention being studied, thereby allowing conclusions regarding the efficacy of the intervention by balancing and "controlling" for other care experiences so that no difference other than the intervention could be responsible for the outcomes. This would include such areas as balance between the groups in office visits and examinations, procedures, experiences, assessments, duration of follow-up and importantly—to the extent possible—experiences with the intervention itself so that no one knows to which intervention an individual study participant is assigned—a topic so important that we will discuss this in a separate section on blinding.

But first—

Important Point: In assessing bias (not just performance bias), some elements of a clinical trial bear scrutiny **both for differences between groups and for their own potential to distort results—** and some may **only bear scrutiny if groups are treated differently.** A good example of an instance where a difference between groups and scrutiny on its own merit is important is duration of study follow-up. Duration may be the same between groups—good for being the same, but bad if too short for patients to experience outcomes. However, let us say that a clinical trial includes a test that you think is completely unnecessary. Because results are derived by **looking at differences in outcomes between groups**, the unnecessary test is generally going to be likely to have no effect on the differences between groups provided it is administered equally. If it is administered disproportionately, however, that could affect outcomes if, say, patients in one group spend more time with a health care practitioner than patients in the comparison group. Remember that our overarching question that guides our entire reading of a study is this: **Can anything explain the study results other than truth? In other words, what caused the outcome?**

Blinding

"Double blinding," "single blinding," "triple blinding"—there is some inconsistency in the way these terms are used—and we don't really care because any opportunity for anyone involved in the research to know the treatment assignment for a study participant can be a problem. So let's keep it simple and just talk about blinding.

Blinding is an important area for critical appraisal assessment. For example, patient and researcher expectations can affect reported study results. Evaluators look for effective blinding for all study subjects and all working with subjects and their data, including blinded assessment. Some areas of examination are, "Who is blinded, how are they blinded, and was the blind likely to be successful?" Inadequately blinded studies have reported distortion of results up to a relative 72 percent, and inadequate blinding of outcomes assessors has been shown to distort results as high as 69 percent.

For example, if patients or study personnel know which patients are receiving the "new" medication or intervention being studied, expectations may be high, and behaviors of patients and those working with patients or patients' data may be affected in such a way as to affect the study outcomes. For example, if it is known that a patient is not getting an active agent, the physician might not care for that patient in the same way, maybe unconsciously providing lesser care, believing that the patient is not going to get better because the patient is not getting an "effective" drug. Or the patient might behave differently in ways that have an impact on the outcomes experienced.

Lack of blinding can affect how outcomes are assessed. If a radiologist is reviewing my x-ray to determine if a tumor is smaller, that assessor might unconsciously (or even consciously) be biased to think my tumor shrank because of knowing that I was being treated with a new chemotherapy agent.

Blinding can even matter when studying objective outcomes such as mortality. The RECORD trial (Rosiglitazone Evaluated for Cardiac Outcomes and Regulation of Glycemia in Diabetes) is an example of an unblinded or open-label trial with blinded assessment in which lack of blinding led to a suspected biased mortality assessment that appears to have significantly altered results. It was determined that event rates for myocardial infarction in the control group were unexpectedly low, which led to an independent review by the FDA which identified myriad problems with case report forms created prior to any blind assessment [Psaty]. The FDA review resulted in a re-analysis [Marciniak], using the available readjudicated case information with the end result that the outcome of non-significance for risk of MI in the original study report changed to a statistically significant difference, the results of which were "remarkably close to results" reported in the original meta-analysis that raised concerns about rosiglitazone and cardiovascular risk in the first place [Nissen].

Critical appraisers are often attentive to looking at who was blinded and how the blinding was accomplished, but then neglect the critical thinking part of the assessment by neglecting to gauge the likelihood that the blind was successful. The attempt to blind a trial when a study group is taking a chemotherapeutic agent with high toxicity and visible effects such as hair loss is going to be unlikely to be successful against a placebo comparator.

List 2. Relative Distortion of Study Results Associated With Blinding

Inadequate Double Blinding—estimated range unclear* to 72%

Juni 01 PMID: 11440947
Kjaergard 01 PMID: 11730399
Moher 98 PMID: 9746022
Savovic 12 PMID: 22945832
Schulz 95 PMID: 7823387

*Savovic 12 PMID 22945832 found in a study of 1,973 trials up to 35% distortion if the endpoint was subjective or mixed, 21% overall, but unclear distortion if the endpoint was mortality or other objective endpoint.

Inadequate Blinding of Assessors—estimated range 35% to 69%

Juni 99 PMID: 10493204
Poolman 07 PMID: 17332104

Clinical Context and Differing Care Experiences

All health care interventions take place within a treatment context where patient and clinician factors such as beliefs, hopes, interactions and previous experiences, along with other aspects of the health care environment may affect study results. The nature and frequency of contacts, quality of communication, degree of empathy, demeanor of practitioners and the amount of reassurance and encouragement provided by clinicians may also affect study results. These factors may, in turn, be affected by blinding. The type of intervention and comparison intervention and how they are experienced by study subjects may also be important factors. For example, the equipment used and method of administering interventions (e.g., injection of medication versus pill) may affect patients' perceptions of efficacy.

Placebo interventions are designed to simulate and balance therapeutic contexts. When an active treatment and placebo are optimally administered in a blinded fashion, the differences in outcomes are likely to be the result of the intervention because the context has been made similar in both groups. The following case study illustrates how differences in care experiences can affect results.

Differences in care experiences frequently occur in non-blinded studies, and these differences may impact patient outcomes. For example, in a single-blinded trial of sham acupuncture in irritable bowel syndrome (IBS) in which blinding appeared to be successful, the investigators disaggregated the placebo effect into two components: 1) a "placebo ritual" alone (placebo acupuncture with needle retracting into the acupuncture needle handle with minimal patient-practitioner interaction); and, 2) placebo ritual plus an "augmented" patient–practitioner relationship [Kaptchuk]. The augmented patient-clinician relationship consisted of attention, warmth, active listening (e.g., repeating patients' words), confidence (e.g., "I have had much positive experience treating IBS and look forward to demonstrating that acupuncture is a valuable treatment in this trial."), and empathy (e.g., "I can understand how IBS can make your usual day more difficult."). Outcomes in each group were compared to outcomes in a third group, a "waiting list" group (no contact with study personnel other than assessments was permitted).

At 3 weeks, the primary outcome measure—adequate relief of IBS symptoms—was reported by 62 percent of participants in the placebo ritual plus supportive care group, 44 percent in the placebo ritual alone group and 28 percent in the usual care (waiting list) group; P<0.001 for each comparison. The results were similar with three other validated measures for irritable bowel syndrome used in the study, and outcomes were similar after an additional 3 weeks of follow-up. The psychosocial context of the care experience, (e.g., the supportive interaction with a practitioner) may be a potent component of treatment effects in some clinical settings.

Differences in Co-interventions Between Groups

Differences in co-interventions in the groups being studied is another area that should be carefully examined in the second area of clinical trials. Allowing use of non-study medications and other interventions may potentially affect the overall study results. This becomes an even more serious problem when such co-interventions become unbalanced between groups.

As an example, in one trial a fixed-dose combination of perindopril and indapamide was compared to placebo, and the primary outcome measure was major microvascular or macrovascular events [Patel]. However, this study was confounded by allowing concomitant therapy at the discretion of the treating physician. Eligible patients were assigned to receive an angiotensin-converting enzyme (ACE) inhibitor, perindopril, in combination with the diuretic, indapamide, or they were assigned to placebo. All other drugs already being taken (except for another ACE inhibitor or thiazide diuretic) were continued, and other non-study antihypertensive drugs could be added during the study. By the end of the trial, more participants assigned to placebo were taking an angiotensin-receptor blocker or a beta blocker, a calcium antagonist, a thiazide, another diuretic or other antihypertensive medication than were those in the intervention group. And by the end of the study, 55 percent of the patients in the control group were taking perindopril.

Allowing the unregulated administration of concomitant medications in a clinical trial creates a risk of a major confounding effect because it has the potential for creating significant differences between the groups. In the example above, it is impossible to tell what was actually responsible for the results. Even though there was a "placebo" control group, the groups were unbalanced by the various combinations of additional antihypertensive medications taken by study participants. We do not know whether the difference in outcomes between the groups was due to active treatment or the co-interventions which differed markedly in the two groups.

~~~

Step 3. Data Collection & Loss of Data—Evaluating a Clinical Trial for Measurement & Attrition Bias

2 Essential Questions for Assessing Measurement & Attrition Bias

1. What information was collected, and how was it collected?

2. What data are missing (e.g., missed measurements, missing patients, were patients unable to complete their course of treatment?), and do missing data meaningfully distort the study results?

What information was collected, and how was it collected?

The third stage in clinical trials is all about data. Measurement is limited not only by what a researcher chooses to measure, but whether something is measurable and whether it was measured correctly. It is important to know if the researcher reported on what he or she measured—or is there the possibility of selective reporting bias?

Selective reporting bias may occur when researchers completely omit reporting of an outcome of interest. At times, it may be important to compare all prespecified outcomes against reported results—and may be worth reviewing the study protocol.

Important omissions can also happen in various ways such as when study design or analysis methods exclude an outcome of interest, which can occur as a partial or complete exclusion. Some deaths appear to have been omitted from the RECORD trial that we already mentioned, due to blinding problems. When we cover time-to-event analyses, we will give you an example of a censoring rule in the APPROVe trial that partially excluded deaths and discuss its impact.

Omission can take another direction as when researchers studying mortality and hormone replacement therapy used only clinical trials in their meta-analysis in which at least one death was reported, thereby inflating mortality outcomes because of not including studies in which no deaths had occurred.

The methods and instruments used for measurement should be evaluated even if the study investigators have stated that their measurement methodology has been "validated." Validation can simply mean that the investigators believe that the measurement methods make sense (face validity), that the methods include the correct items (content validity) and that the measurement methods are accurate and dependable (construct validity). Even if a data collection instrument has earned the label of "validated," it might actually not be an appropriate instrument for the study in question. It may, in fact, not be valid at all. Obviously judgment is involved in these three validation areas, and the third of these—accuracy and dependability—requires a valid measurement method for comparison. Appraisers will need to make their own judgments about the validity of the measurement methods which might entail performing a critical appraisal of the evidence regarding a measurement instrument and its validation study as part of a critical appraisal assessment for a clinical trial.

As a practical matter, we may seek out information, frequently from a specialist, about the standard instruments used to address specific questions. If we find the researcher is using an instrument that is not considered a standard, then we may go to the extra effort of critically appraising research on that instrument.

Missing data are also an important critical appraisal consideration, which leads to attrition bias—

What data are missing and do missing data meaningfully distort the study results?

Attrition bias is generally thought of as "loss of subjects to follow-up." However, we believe the issue is a larger one and can pretty much be simplified by asking what data are missing. Considerations include how much information was lost, when it was lost, why it was lost and whether this loss is likely to have meaningfully affected results.

There are thousands of studies about the effect of various biases on research outcomes. However, the effect of attrition on distortion of study results has been the least clear. Consequently, many in the research community struggle with this area. List 3 shows some evidence on this and illustrates the large range of estimated distortion of results that might occur due to attrition bias.

List 3. Relative Distortion of Study Results in Clinical Trials Associated with Data Collection & Attrition Bias

Loss of Data (Attrition Bias)—estimated range 2 to 38%

COTS 07 PMID: 17200303
Nuesch 09 PMID: 19736281
Tierney 04 PMID: 15561753
van Tulder 09 PMID: 19770609

Completer Analysis—estimated range 56% with 44% early withdrawal

Shih 02 PMID: 11985778

Assessment Models for Missing Data—with loss of 20% risk of type I error* is approximately 10%; with loss of 40% risk of type I is approximately 50%

Lachin 00 PMID: 11018568

* *Type 1 - or alpha error - A difference is reported, but there is no difference (i.e., a false positive).*

Frequently, approaches are taken which put a cap on accepting a certain amount of attrition. For example, some journals have capped acceptable attrition at 20 percent. However, attrition is not the same as attrition bias, and the real question is whether or not attrition bias is present and, if yes, has it meaningfully distorted results? Using a cap is likely to result in rejecting some otherwise reliable studies. For these reasons, we favor an approach that looks at the contextual elements of studies on a case-by-case basis.

Consider, we are seeking truth (cause and effect). Also, consider that we are always testing interventions on a sample of the population. If the intervention works, and if we had a sufficient number of people to actually experience the events of interest, it may not matter if we have less than half of the population we started out with, for example. Truth should be the same no matter how large or small our population is if we have enough people to show a true difference in a valid study.

For any given study with two arms, there are four possibilities. In a two-arm study, either—

1. Intervention A > Intervention B

2. Intervention A < Intervention B

3. Intervention A = Intervention B

4. And/or another intervention affects results

And so our approach is to try to understand these questions: What would be required for any possible scenario to be true? Were those conditions met? What is the likelihood of reported outcomes to be distorted by bias or explained by chance? Are there clues to the likely true answer?

In examining this, it is important to be aware that study outcomes are due to either bias or chance, or study results are true. Because of the challenges that safety presents, we are focusing on efficacy results from superiority trials.

One starting point for us is to look closely at study design, methodology and execution because a well-designed and well-executed study may protect against attrition bias even when attrition is high.

Many study factors have an impact on attrition bias, and successful blinding frequently is one of the most important elements. To illustrate this, let's imagine a study in which patients are on an active agent or placebo. And now let us imagine that care was not taken to conceal assignment of patients to their study groups. A physician who knows his or her patient is on placebo might be more likely to be impatient about treatment outcomes and encourage a patient to seek other treatment as compared to a physician who knows his or her patient is receiving the active agent. Therefore, the resulting attrition would be due to bias and not necessarily due to the effect of the study agent and, in this example, the results may be meaningfully distorted if a sufficient number of physicians acted in this manner and patients complied, a bias would be created. Examples of this problem have appeared in the medical literature.

A second starting point for us is to look closely at various study performance outcomes (such as the likely success of blinding, treatment adherence or reasons for discontinuation) and study results as there may be informative clues as to whether meaningful attrition bias is present or as to which of the possible scenarios is most likely to be true.

For example, it is important to review the reasons for discontinuation. If many more patients in one group are seeking active treatment, depending upon certain study quality features, this may point to lack of effect. However, it's important to keep in mind that this could be an incorrect assumption because the seeking of another treatment could be the result of a bias such as in our earlier example of the unblinded physicians.

So if you have a study in which you have a balanced baseline, no planned differences between groups except for what is being studied, and in which blinding is likely to have been successful, then here is our advice for other areas to look at to consider whether or not attrition has resulted in meaningful attrition bias.

Look for informative patterns (e.g., relatedness of outcomes)

Equality OR inequality may be informative such as in the following 5 examples:

1. Exposure (e.g., adherence, protocol violations, duration)

2. Baseline characteristics of all subjects by group compared to baseline characteristics of completers by group

3. Number and reasons for discontinuations by group

4. Examine co-interventions for likelihood of a superior co-intervention, balance or imbalance (or likely imbalance) between groups, and potential to meaningfully distort results

5. Censoring rules that might result in a potential for bias between groups ("censoring" is the practice of removing a subject from a survival curve)

Would any sensitivity analyses help answer the question?

Assess likelihood of chance

Are there confirmatory high quality studies?

When it comes to attrition and the potential for attrition bias to meaningfully affect the results, there can be a tremendous interplay among many study elements.

It is also important to keep in mind that when there are gaps in data, sometimes authors use models, and models rely on assumptions which may be invalid or unverifiable. Frequently, such assumptions are not reported in articles.

~~~

Step 4. Assessing The Differences In The Outcomes Of The Study Groups—Evaluating a Clinical Trial for Assessment Bias

2 Essential Questions for Assessing Assessment Bias

1. How is the difference in outcomes between the groups evaluated?

2. What are those differences, and how are they expressed?

We already shared with you that we're not going to go deeply into statistical methods. If we have a concern about statistical methods, we may do a little research about the methods or seek out a statistician for a consult. Rarely do we take this latter step. We have evaluated thousands of studies and have felt we needed to seek such advice only a handful of times.

What we will cover here, however, are **a few analysis methods** and a **few simple but important statistics.**

1. How is the difference in outcomes between the groups evaluated?

Intention-to-Treat (ITT) Analysis

For dichotomous outcomes of efficacy in superiority trials, ITT analysis is historically considered by many journal editors to be a favored analysis method (i.e., CONSORT Statement history). ITT analysis requires that patients are analyzed in the group to which they are randomized regardless of the actual intervention received and regardless of study completion or completeness of data, which requires the use of some reasonable method for assigning missing data points (data imputation).

Important Note 1: ITT analysis is not appropriate for analyzing safety outcomes because it could mask important safety information.

Important Note 2: ITT is not appropriate for non-inferiority and equivalence trials if the data imputation methods favor no difference between groups, which is generally the case.

Having said that, ITT analysis would seem to be a peculiar method to favor when we are trying to discover truth. However, ITT analysis is an attempt to try and minimize some problems that can result when patients inadvertently receive an unassigned intervention or when data are missing. By requiring that patients are analyzed as randomized, ITT analysis is an attempt to preserve the benefits of randomization. By requiring that every patient be accounted for by including a value for each patient, ITT analysis is an attempt to mitigate problems arising from missing data.

It's easy to tell if ITT analysis has been performed. The number randomized to each group should equal the number analyzed in each group—and they should be the same people.

An area that is a bit more complex is evaluating the data imputation. There are two frequently used approaches for imputing missing data. The first method attempts to estimate "truth." The second method attempts to set a bar for reaching statistical significance. We, ourselves, employ this second method to do our own analyses when facing the situation of an otherwise valid study that is doomed to receive an "uncertainty" grade from us without this kind of analysis.

Imputation Methods Approximating Truth

Methods which attempt to approximate the truth include—

- Mixed effects models (e.g., mixed linear, two-stage random effects or random coefficient models), multiple imputation models and a cumulative change approach. A reminder that these are models, models are not truth, and assumptions used in creating models are infrequently reported and so usually cannot be evaluated. That said, many statisticians favor this method when attempting to approximate the truth, and so we tend to be accepting of these methods. However, we may take a close look at attrition as we have described above to discern how big an impact modeling may have on the outcomes.

- LOCF (last-observation-carried-forward) is prone to bias and should usually not be used. However, in some situations when the study is of a progressive condition in which overall improvement could not be expected to happen without some kind of effective intervention, LOCF may be conservative and reasonable at least to determine the direction of the outcomes (e.g., efficacy). This, however, depends upon meeting certain validity requirements as described here:

  http://www.delfini.org/delfiniClick_PrimaryStudies.htm#LOCFhelp.

- For readers who wish further information regarding LOCF, the following two references will be of value [Carpenter, O'Brien].

- Baseline-carried-forward may be a possibly acceptable method under certain circumstances. The key is to think through what the likely effect on outcomes might be.

Imputation Methods for Challenging the Data

These methods usually employ conservative approaches to fill in missing data gaps for the purpose of determining at what point outcomes are no longer statistically significant.

The easiest method to describe is "extreme-case analysis." This method puts the intervention under study through the toughest test possible. For example, an extreme-case analysis might count all missing patients in the intervention group as "treatment failures" and all missing patients in the placebo group as "treatment successes." If the difference between the groups remains statistically significant after this test in an otherwise valid study, we can be fairly confident that the intervention has proved the direction of the outcomes, even if we do not know with accuracy the effect size.

However, surviving an extreme-case analysis is a pretty tall order, requiring a perfect combination of effect size and amount of missing data. Therefore, we usually apply some kind of variation. We might start with extreme-case analysis in case we get lucky, and then ratchet the numbers downward until we can find the breaking point for statistical significance. We then look at the resulting outcome and then decide whether we think our test has been reasonable.

Another method that we frequently use is to assign the recovery rate of those in the placebo group (also known as the "control event rate") for missing values in both groups and then test the statistical significance in outcomes between groups.

Another example is documented in a study of prehypertension in which missing patients in both the candesartan and the placebo group were counted as failed. Since blood pressure is unlikely to spontaneously improve from anything active in the placebo (in that both the placebo and the study drug could account for placebo effect), this appears to have been a reasonable choice [Julius 06].

What becomes especially challenging is how to decide what is "conservative" when two or more active agents are being compared.

Evaluating the method used for data imputation is critically important because how the imputation is done can dramatically affect not only effect size, but potentially also the direction of the results. (And this is an area that we see critical appraisers routinely ignore.)

We're always happy to see additional kinds of analyses performed, such as completer analyses, but even with its limitations, we find ITT analysis frequently helpful and informative particularly if done conservatively.

Time-to-Event (TTE) Analysis

Time-to-event analyses are methods to evaluate the length of time to an outcome of interest such as time-to-cancer progression or time-to-pregnancy. Related terms include life table analysis and survival analysis which refer to the method regardless of whether survival is the outcome. Kaplan-Meier (KM) methodology is the most commonly used survival analysis in health care research.

Time-to-event, or TTE, analysis, is a complex area, so only a few key points will be made here. A key point is that censoring may or may not increase the risk of bias in a TTE analysis. Again, censoring can be defined as removing a patient's data from a TTE at a certain time in the trial. Investigators censor patients for multiple reasons.

For example, because a time-to-event bias could result from subjects spending different amounts of time in the study, some patient data are typically excluded from the analysis. This is one type of "censoring" also referred to as "right-censoring" or "administrative censoring" and is not considered to be biased provided that groups are balanced in terms of timing of patients being enrolled in the study. Randomization automatically takes care of this.

However, investigators can create any other kinds of censoring rules they desire—and so you can imagine why it is important to evaluate them as some choices may be highly prone to bias.

Results of TTE analyses are generally reported as graphs on a "curve" which is actually a series of steps. This series of steps is called a Kaplan Meier curve or a survival curve. The curves are created through a mathematical calculation which creates a drop in a line each time an event occurs, and censored patients are also removed from the calculation. (Frequently, TTE analyses are reported as "using the ITT principle," but this really isn't a true application of ITT analysis because of the censored data as compared to ITT analysis which requires analyzing a full data set.)

Data censoring can create some of the biggest problems in TTE analysis. An important critical appraisal issue is that inappropriate censoring may distort a curve.

- KM models assume on average that the likelihood of experiencing an endpoint is the same for early-enrolled subjects as well as for subjects enrolled later—and this may not be a valid assumption.
- KM models assume that the likelihood of experiencing an endpoint is the same for censored and non-censored patients— and this too may not be a valid assumption.
- Frequently the reasons for censoring are not reported, which makes it impossible for critical appraisers to assess the censoring for bias.
- Censored data are assumed to occur randomly, which may not be a valid assumption.
- Data for censored patients are not included after the point subjects are censored, which could distort results.
- Censoring reduces sample size, which may reduce reliability of results.
- Censored subjects may differ from subjects remaining in the study, which may create bias.

Assessing the potential for bias in TTE analyses is important. Researchers have reported that problems with TTE analysis may misrepresent outcomes by a relative 50 percent or higher [Lachin 00]. However, it is frequently the case that insufficient information about censoring is provided by researchers. Critical appraisers need to know information about the number of censored patients, the timing of censoring and reasons for censoring.

Let us tell you a little story. Again, we return to Vioxx. In one of the Vioxx studies, for one of their analyses, investigators decided that they would censor any patients who experienced a confirmed thrombotic event 14 days after ceasing study medication under the assumption that the harm could not be a result of the medication. This decision resulted in a radically different point at which the divergence of the curves was statistically significant as compared to not applying this censoring rule.

Such a rule should never have been applied. If it was true that the harm was not a result of study medication, that would have been revealed through a comparison between the two groups. Luckily, this biased censoring rule was discovered by a reader who published a re-analysis after putting the missing patients back into the analysis [Mundell], with the result that many more lawsuits over blood clots due to Vioxx occurred.

We have rarely seen censoring rules reported in studies. At times we are able to obtain that information by reviewing the protocol or other supplementary information or by contacting the researchers. When we are unable to get this information, if a study is otherwise valid, we frequently try to assess the validity of outcomes through other means such as doing our own intention-to-treat analysis, if possible, or assessing patterns in outcomes reported in different ways.

2. What are those differences, and how are they expressed?

Here come the statistics! We will present very few, and these will be easy. "Measures of outcomes" are statistics that show the size of differences between the results of the study groups. Some synonyms for measures of outcomes include "measures of association" and "measures of risk." Measures of outcomes can be used to express a variety of things such as probability or odds of benefit or harm or the number of people needed to be screened to benefit a person, the number needed to prevent an untoward outcome and so on.

Measures of outcomes represent what is called the "effect size" meaning the difference in size of outcomes between the groups studied. Some other synonyms for effect size include "estimates of effect," "point estimates" and "treatment effect."

There are various measures of outcomes.

There are those which are natural frequencies. These include risk with and without treatment and number-out-of-100.

There are probability measures such as—

- Absolute Risk Reduction or the ARR

- Number-Needed-to-Treat, known as the NNT

- Relative Risk or RR

- Relative Risk Reduction or the RRR

These measures often have a complementary measure. Absolute risk increase (ARI) is the complement to absolute risk reduction (ARR). Number-needed-to-harm is the complement to number-needed-to-treat (NNT).

There are many ratios which describe various outcomes when the results of two or more groups are being compared. The three most commonly encountered ratios are odds ratio, relative risk ratio (almost always referred to as relative risk or, less frequently, risk ratio) and hazard ratio. Hazard ratios are measures used to compare outcomes in groups when time-to-event analyses, such as Kaplan-Meier models, are used.

Measures of Outcomes and Time

Measures of outcomes should always be associated with a time period and, with rare exception, that time period is the study time period. There is a big difference in a headache medication that rids you of your migraine in an hour as compared to one that takes a full day. So this time period may be additionally important information in assessing meaningful clinical benefit. However, it is hard to assess exactly when benefit is obtained and so the time period is usually expressed as being "within" the study time period.

Description of Various Measures of Outcomes

The Natural Frequencies: Risk With and Without Treatment

Risk with and without treatment is simply the observed number of outcomes in each group expressed as the number who experienced an outcome and the number who did not. For example, it might be that 10 people out of 100 in the intervention group died compared to 15 out of 100 in the placebo group. This method of expressing the difference between groups provides the most useful and complete information, which we illustrate when we describe absolute risk reduction.

This is also the information that is used to create what is referred to as a 2-by-2 table. A 2-by-2 table is used to compute many important statistics such as p-values and confidence intervals.

Risk With and Without Treatment Summary
Control group: 10 out of 100 improve
Study group: 15 out of 100 improve

That's it!

Absolute Risk Reduction (ARR)

In addition to knowing risk with and without treatment, it is helpful to know the absolute risk reduction or the ARR. Absolute risk reduction is expressed as a percentage and is simply computed by subtracting the percentage of patients experiencing the outcome in each group.

In the above example, 15 percentage points minus 10 percentage points provides us with an absolute risk reduction of 5 percent. As you can see, knowing a 5 percent difference is not as meaningful as knowing risk with and without treatment as well.

Consider, a patient might make a very different decision about taking a medication in the following two scenarios.

Control group = 90 out of 100 die; intervention group = 85 out of 100 die. I am highly likely to die. I am willing to take great risk in the hopes that I will be one of the lucky 5 percent that survives.

Control group =15 out of 100 die; intervention group = 10 out of 100 die. I consider my risk of death low no matter what choice I make. I am willing to risk that I am not one of the 5 percent who will benefit and so wish to forego the medication and its potential harms and cost.

ARR Summary
Control group: 10 out of 100 improve
Study group: 15 out of 100 improve
ARR = 5%
In this example, ARR (the actual difference between groups as a percent) is 15% minus 10% = 5%.

This means that 5 percent more people who take the study drug will realize improvement as compared to the people who receive the control medication.

Relative Risk Reduction (RRR)

A commonly reported measure of outcome is the relative risk reduction or the RRR. Relative risk reduction is the proportional difference in size between outcomes. So in our example, 10 is one third smaller than 15; one third equals 33 percent. So the RRR is 33 percent. The formula for RRR = [((Comparison group outcomes - Intervention group outcomes) / Comparison group outcomes) x 100]. In this case (15%-5%)/15%=33%. (Note that the RRR can also be obtained by using the formula 1-RR, which stands for relative risk, which we will get to next.)

Mathematically, the relative risk reduction **may equal the absolute risk reduction, but it is never smaller**. In fact, usually it is bigger—

frequently a lot bigger. Our Vioxx example of 60 percent benefit (of less than 1 percent benefit) being an important case in point.

Whenever you see the term "relative" used for a measure of outcome, your question should be "relative to what?"

RRR Summary
Control group: 10 out of 100 improve
Study group: 15 out of 100 improve
RRR = 33%
RRR in this example 15% minus 10% divided by 15% or 33%.

This means that there is a relative 33 percent improvement for those people who take the study drug as compared to the people who receive the control medication.

Relative Risk (RR)

Relative risk provides readers with an estimate of the risk of some health-related event, such as disease or death, when compared to one or more comparison groups. Relative risk is expressed as the number of times one group may be at risk over another. A relative risk of less than 1 represents a lower risk than the comparison group. The formula for RR = risk in study group outcomes divided by risk in the comparison group. (Again, note that the RRR can also be obtained by using the formula 1-RR.)

RR Summary
Control group: 10 out of 100 improve
Intervention group: 15 out of 100 improve
Risk in control group: 10%
Risk in intervention group: 15%
RR in this example is 10%/15% = 2/3 or 67%

This means that people in the intervention group have a reduced risk of 67 percent as compared to the people who receive the control medication.

Odds and Odds Ratios (OR)

In many single studies, you will be dealing with probability measures such as absolute and relative risk reduction. But it also is helpful to understand other measures that are more typically used in other kinds of studies. Odds are similar to probability, but slightly different. In the case of odds, we will give you an example first, and then we will give you the explanation: because of having 13 cards in each of 4 suits, the odds of drawing an ace in a standard poker playing deck of 52 cards is 4/48 or 1/12; however, the probability of drawing an ace is 4/52 or 1/13.

Odds represent the likelihood of an event occurring compared to not occurring. For example, the odds of two to one mean that likelihood of an event occurring is twice that of not occurring. This differs from probability where the numerator contains the number of times the event occurs, but the denominator contains the number of times the event could have occurred. **Odds and probabilities of outcomes are similar if the event rate is low.**

Odds ratios are employed in case-control studies to quantify a mathematical relationship between an exposure and a health outcome. Odds are used in case-control studies because the investigator arbitrarily controls the study populations (i.e., creates denominators for the calculations). Odds ratios are calculated by dividing the odds in the exposed case by the odds in the control case. Odds are often used in other types of studies as well, such as meta-analysis, because of various properties of odds which have some advantages for computing purposes mathematically.

OR Summary

Odds represent the likelihood of an event occurring compared to not occurring. Odds ratios are calculated by dividing the odds in the one study group by the odds in the other group.

Investigators in a case-control study report that 20/100 subjects in the control group die and 10/100 subjects in the treatment group die:

Odds of death in control group = 20/80 = 25%
Odds of death in treatment group = 10/90 = 11%
Odds ratio = 0.25/0.11 = 2.27.

This means that the odds of dying are about 2+ times greater for people in the control group as compared to the people who receive the treatment.

Number-needed-to-treat (NNT)

Number-needed-to-treat, or the NNT, is the reciprocal of the absolute risk reduction—meaning you are just taking the absolute risk reduction out of being a percentage by dividing the ARR into 100.

For an absolute risk reduction of 5 percent, you take the number of the percent—5 in our ARR example above—and divide 100 by that number. Five goes into 100 twenty times, so the NNT is 20. So that means for an absolute risk reduction of 5 percent, you have to treat 20 patients to benefit one person within the study timeframe as compared to the comparison treatment.

NNT Summary

Placebo group: 10 out of 100 improve
Study group: 15 out of 100 improve
ARR = 5%
NNT = 20, meaning that out of every 20 patients treated with the study drug, 1 more person will experience a benefit than if they were treated with placebo within the study time period.

The Natural Frequencies: Number-out-of-100

For the natural frequency of number-out-of-100, take the number of the percent—in this example, 5—which would then be 5 out of 100 patients would benefit within the study time period as compared to the comparison treatment.

Hazard Rates and Hazard Ratios (HR)

For time-to-event analyses, hazard rates and hazard ratios are used. A hazard is an incidence rate. A hazard represents the likelihood of a patient who has not experienced the outcome of interest, experiencing an event at a specific point on a Kaplan-Meier curve (i.e., meaning at a particular point in time on the curve). A hazard rate—or the slope of the survival curve—is a measure of how rapidly subjects in one group are experiencing the endpoint.

A hazard ratio approximates the relative risk in the intervention group compared to the control group. Hazard ratios use regression models to calculate rates in time-to-event analyses. For most readers it may be most useful to think of hazard ratios as the chance of an event occurring in the treatment arm divided by the chance of the event occurring in the control arm, or vice versa, of a study.

For example, with an HR of two, a patient who has not yet experienced the outcome at a certain time has twice the chance of experiencing the outcome at the next point in time compared to a subject in the control group.

An assumption of proportional hazards regression is that the hazard ratio is constant over time. Although this may not be true, the hazard ratio provides useful information regarding the relative likelihood of an event in the treated versus control subjects at any given point in time.

Median survival in each group is usually presented with hazard ratios. Hazard ratios (calculated by software using regression models) are usually presented in the results sections reporting TTE analyses and also with the Kaplan-Meier graphs.

HR Summary

Hazard Ratios approximate the relative risk in the intervention group compared to the control group in a Kaplan-Meier or other time-to-event (TTE) model.

Example: "The time to prostate-specific antigen (PSA) progression was 8.3 months (placebo) vs. 3.0 months (drug A); hazard ratio, 0.25; p<0.001)." In this case, the hazard ratio approximates a 25% relative risk reduction with the drug.

Chance

To have a chance effect in research means that the observed outcomes are not truly due to the intervention, and they are not a result of bias, but rather the findings are a random accident.

Statistical significance (frequently shortened merely to **"significance"** and **not to be confused with clinical significance**), is the term used for a measurement that addresses some unique aspects of the probability of having a chance effect. To determine statistical significance, p-values and confidence intervals are calculated.

P-values are largely misunderstood and are less helpful in evaluating the probability of chance effects than most people think. Here is a technical definition for p-values:

"Assuming there truly is no difference between the groups studied, the p-value is a calculated probability of observing a difference as big as or bigger than the one you observed in a study based on compatibility with an assumed standard distribution."

Consider the following scenario: Drug A is compared to placebo, and there are 100 subjects in each group. Assume that mortality in Drug A group is 5 percent, that mortality in the placebo group is 15 percent, and that the p-value = 0.03. In this scenario, the p-value can be interpreted as follows: "If it is true that there is no difference in mortality outcomes between Drug A and placebo, then there is a 3 percent statistical probability (chance) of observing a difference equal to or greater than the difference represented by 5 deaths out of 100 in the Drug A group as compared to 15 deaths out of 100 in the placebo group."

As you can see, the p-value is actually quite complex, is limited and is built upon assumptions which may not be true. The p-value cannot tell you the chance that the results are true or even how likely they are to be due to chance. Consequently, we don't find p-values and the whole arena of statistical significance to be definitively helpful, but because p-values are frequently misunderstood, they may be frequently relied upon, which is important for you to know.

Our approach is to consider the p-value merely as an indicator of the potential for chance effects. Review of confirmatory studies and patterns are potentially better ways to help address the likelihood of reported study results being due to chance or not.

Statistical Significance

- Statistically significant results are also called **positive outcomes** or positive results, or we may say that the results went in a positive direction. Thus, results can be "positive" for increased mortality because the "positive" refers to positive statistical significance and not whether outcomes are beneficial or harmful.

- A couple of shorthand terms for falsely positive outcomes are alpha- or type I errors: *A difference is reported, but there is no difference.* This can be due to bias, confounding or chance.

- The value at which results will be considered significant should be determined prior to the start of the study. This is called setting the alpha level or setting alpha.

Non-statistically Significant Findings & Power

In **Selection Bias: Are There Enough People**, we shared with you the happy news that most readers can ignore power calculations—but you do need to understand what it means for a study to be "powered"—and happily, it is a very easy concept (but one which is frequently misunderstood).

- Power simply means that, if there is a true difference between groups (i.e., a statistically significant difference), you had enough people to reveal that difference. Therefore, ANY statistically significant difference is *de facto* powered for that outcome.

- If statistical significance is **not** reached for an outcome, it is called a "**negative finding**." However, a negative finding could be a chance effect—even more so than a positive (meaning statistically significant) finding. For example, if no differences were found between groups in a safety outcome, it does not necessarily mean that the drugs studied are equal in safety. **Negative findings always raise a question whether it is true there is no difference between the groups or whether there were simply too few people to show a difference if there truly is one.** ("No difference" is the common parlance for "no statistically significant difference.") In other words, was the outcome underpowered?

- What this means is that you need a sufficient number of people to capture study events, which is dependent upon the frequency of events in that population. (Frequency, not necessarily meaning multiple events per person—although it could.) Frequency could be something such as this: within 1 year, 3 people out of 1,000 will experience a heart attack with no treatment, and 1 person out of 1,000 will experience a heart attack if taking Drug A. If we were studying only 100 people, the likelihood of any event occurring is low and so a difference between the groups might not be discovered.

- Therefore, in this example of a study of Drug A, if we did not have a statistically significant outcome (and *anytime* we do not have a statistically significant outcome), we have two questions: **is it true there is no difference between the groups, or did we just not have enough people to reveal the difference?** In other words, was the study "powered" for that outcome? So to talk about a study being powered is simply shorthand for, "Were there enough people studied to show a statistically significant difference if one truly exists in a particular outcome?"

- And here's where we see a lot of people getting lost in the lingo. **If you reach statistical significance, by definition, you _had_ enough people.** Ergo, the study was powered for that outcome.

- False negative findings are also referred to as type II or beta errors: *No difference is reported, but there is a difference.*

More on Chance

Before a study begins, a decision is made to set the boundary at which the p-value will be considered statistically significant. Frequently, the level of significance is set at less than point 05—or less than 5 percent—although it may be set at much less than that. Less than point 05 was merely set historically as a convention. The p-value is generated by the size of difference in an outcome between groups along with the size of the study population.

A number of things can increase the risk of chance outcomes such as—

- Small sample size,

- Observing outcomes that are not prespecified—"prespecification" is often referred to as *a priori,*

- Analyzing subgroups that are not *a priori,*

- Terminating the study sooner than planned—even if cautionary procedures, called "stopping rules," are applied; and,

- Multiple analyses.

When it comes to multiple analyses, there two big categories that can increase the opportunity for chance effects:

- Performing interim analyses; and,

- Analyzing many outcomes even if they are prespecified.

For example, if researchers decide to set significance at "<0.05" in a study, that means that there is a less than 1 in 20 chance—or less than a 5 percent chance—that an outcome of interest will be found to be statistically significant merely due to chance. Evaluating two outcomes now increases this risk as high as 2 in 20 times.

It is also important to be aware that there is some controversy about the legitimacy of statistically significant secondary outcomes if primary outcomes do not reach significance. Some critical appraisers will not pay any attention to statistically significant secondary outcomes if the primary outcome has not reached significance.

There are others—including ourselves—who do not take this position. We believe it is more important to look at all outcomes studied and see if there are patterns.

Both sides of this controversy have reasonable points, and so there is no good resolution to this issue.

~~~

Evaluating Results: The 5 Clinically Significant Outcomes

Once you've determined that a clinical trial is valid, then comes the task of assessing results. As we've discussed, we actually consider this question even before we evaluate a clinical trial because, unless the results are clinically useful, we are unlikely to be interested in spending our time reviewing the trial.

A key question patients need answered for each therapeutic option before making decisions about their health care is, "What is the likelihood of benefit and harm for me, and what is the quality of the evidence upon which that is based?" We believe there is likely to be no disagreement with the following five hopes all people have:

That we don't die prematurely (mortality).

- That we don't suffer from conditions or diseases that we can avoid (morbidity).

- That we do not experience unpleasant symptoms from our health issues if they cannot be avoided (symptom relief).

- That health issues do not interfere with our daily activities (emotional, physical and mental functioning).

- That our health issues do not detract from our quality of life (health-related quality of life).

This is just another way of talking about what we have already described as the five clinically significant outcomes (morbidity, mortality, symptom relief, functioning and health-related quality of life). If a studied research outcome is not one of these five things, then it is an "intermediate marker." Such surrogates are "assumed" to stand in for clinically meaningful outcomes, but may not as we have explained above.

Knowing that an intervention provides better results than the comparison intervention, we then need to understand the difference between the groups. We've discussed the various measures of outcomes already. We also find it very helpful to look at confidence intervals. If the investigators have not provided you with the confidence intervals, frequently you can easily calculate these yourself. There are many easy-to-use confidence interval calculators available online, and we list some on our website at our recommended web links.

Confidence Intervals (CIs)

A confidence interval is a calculation of a range of possible results that are statistically as plausible as the true calculation observed in the study. They can be computed for any measure of outcome. For example, if a study is very small—meaning if the study has a very small subject population—and we observed 8 deaths in the placebo group, but only 5 in the intervention group, it is more likely that the reported outcomes are a chance effect, and we would learn more about what is truly to be expected if we had more people in the study. So, if we had more study subjects, we might be more likely to see a much smaller difference or a much larger difference. So the confidence interval might tell us that minus 20 to positive 23 are equally plausible statistically to the observed actual difference of 3.

A 95 percent confidence interval means that the calculation provides for a 5 percent range of chance that the true population value lies outside the calculated confidence interval range. If the calculation were set at 90 percent, that would mean the range for chance was established at 10 percent, and so on.

It is important to note that confidence intervals are built on the same assumptions as p-values and so have similar limitations.

That said, the confidence interval has many uses and is more helpful to evaluate than p-values. We find confidence intervals useful because they can help to quantify uncertainty by providing a range (e.g., the wider the range, the greater the uncertainty), they can assist with assessing meaningful clinical benefit, and they can help to deal with conclusivity of non-significant findings (Type II or beta error). But an important thing to note is that studies have shown that the most likely answer in a valid study to actually be most accurate is the actual calculated result observed in the study.

CI Summary

Example:
Placebo group: 10 out of 100 improve
Study group: 15 out of 100 improve

Example 1: If ARR = 5%, **95% CI** (-4.14% to 14.14%), this means that, given a 5% play of chance, the population value is estimated between -4.14% and 14.14%.

Example 2: If ARR = 5%, **90% CI** (-2.67% to 12.67%), this means that, given a 10% play of chance, the population value is estimated between -2.67% and 12.67%.

We will add one other little tip about confidence intervals. Confidence intervals can be used to ascertain whether or not an effect size is statistically significant or not. To do so, you need to remember one little trick.

When No Difference is Zero: "No difference" for those effect sizes which are expressed as percentages = 0. So for measures of outcomes such as ARR or RRR, you look to see if the confidence intervals pass through zero. In the above examples, we can see that the outcomes are not statistically significant.

When No Difference Is One: "No difference" for those effect sizes which are expressed as ratios = 1. (A helpful aid to memory is to keep in mind that, in a ratio, a 1-to-1 correspondence is "no difference.") So for measures of outcomes such as OR or RR, you look to see if the confidence intervals pass through one.

Using CIs to Establish Meaningful Clinical Outcomes

For statistically significant results, is the confidence interval wholly within your judgment for meaningful clinical benefit? Example: You decide you want to see at least a 1 percent reduction in mortality—this is a judgment. *Your* judgment. If the study reports an absolute risk reduction, or an ARR of 2, 95% CI (1 to 3), this meets your requirement for meaningful clinical benefit and, therefore, as a practical measure, these results can be considered conclusive (given a 5% margin for the play of chance, which we derived by subtracting the chosen level for the confidence interval—in this instance 95%—from 100 percent).

Using CIs to "Practically" Evaluate the Potential Reliability of Non-significant Findings

Findings that are not statistically significant raise the very important question: **Is there truly no difference between the groups?** Or was the study size too small to detect a difference. We refer to this as the study being insufficiently powered for that particular outcome in question (i.e., type II or beta error).

Confidence intervals come in handy when facing non-significant findings. As a practical approach, you can look at the confidence intervals and, if the interval includes what you would consider to be a clinically meaningful difference, then you may decide that the study results are inconclusive. If the interval excludes any value that you would consider clinically significant, then as a practical matter it is reasonable to conclude that there is no meaningful difference between the groups.

Example 1: You decide you want to see at least a 4 percent reduction in mortality—this is a judgment. *Your* judgment. If the study reports an absolute risk reduction, or an ARR of 2, 95% CI (1 to 3), this does not meet your requirement for meaningful clinical benefit, and so it is reasonable for you to conclude, as a practical matter, that there is no clinically meaningful difference between the groups even though the results are actually statistically significant.

Example 2: You decide that 3 percent bleeding in use of anti-coagulation medications after hip replacement surgery is clinically meaningful to you. Again, this is your judgment. If the study reports an absolute risk increase, or an ARI of 2, 95% CI (-2 to 4), this includes the potential for what you deem to be clinically meaningful bleeding, and so it is reasonable for you to conclude, as a practical matter, that it is inconclusive that there is no difference between the groups even though the reported outcomes are not statistically significant.

~~~

Safety

Safety issues concern risks and harms which are events that cause problems with meaningful outcomes (morbidity, mortality, adverse symptoms, reduction in health-related quality of life, diminished functioning) or cause other unwanted effects. Harms represent a challenge to evaluate for many reasons. They are usually infrequent. They are usually not the focus of study. They are rarely determined *a priori* and, therefore, there is a greater likelihood that differences in safety outcomes are due to chance. Many trials do not fully report adverse events. Many trials are of insufficient duration to detect harms or are of insufficient size to detect differences between groups. As we have discussed, a common mistake is to conclude that statistically non-significant differences in adverse events are due to no difference in interventions when in fact the trial was not powered to detect the differences. Non-significant differences between groups could be chance effects, could be due to insufficient numbers of patients to find differences between groups—or could truly be due to no difference between groups. High discontinuation rates in studies may result in agents appearing safer than they actually are.

For all of the above reasons, we must look for harms that are reported from weaker science such as case report data, database research, observational studies, registries or low quality clinical trials. At the same time we must remember that, if outcome measures are not identified *a priori*, it increases the possibility that the findings are due to chance and that low quality evidence is likely to give us incorrect results. There are many examples where effective interventions are no longer available (e.g., have been discontinued by the manufacturer) due to incorrect safety data. When this happens, patients may suffer if reasonable alternatives are not available.

It is unlikely that a reader can draw safety conclusions from a single clinical trial unless the trial is extremely large and of high quality and/or if the rate of harm appears to be meaningfully different between the groups. Even if the reader obtains systematic reviews of clinical trials dealing with harms, they may not be detected if some of the included trials do not report harms or if harms are described in various ways in different studies. In some cases, systematic reviews may falsely indicate lack of harms that are subsequently detected in large, well-designed and -conducted RCTs. For a rigorous assessment of harms, critical appraisers should include assessments of clinical trials, systematic reviews and observational studies such as those from registries, keeping in mind that observational studies are prone to bias and that these efforts may still miss important safety information.

Readers should also remember that in clinical trials, the **safety population should *only* be those who receive the intervention** (for drugs, this should be all patients receiving at least one dose of a study medication). For safety, patients should be **analyzed *by their intervention assignment* and not as randomized**.

As we have described, confidence intervals are extremely helpful in evaluating harms in clinical trials. Unless a study is powered for harms, lack of statistically significant differences may mean there is no difference or it may mean it is still unknown if there is a difference. Review of confidence intervals (CIs) of non-significant findings to discern if there is a clinically meaningful difference between the groups within the confidence interval provides important information, as we have pointed out.

When we evaluate harms, we find it useful to review multiple clinical trials and other studies looking for patterns of harms. We note if support exists for the existence of the harm (e.g., biologic plausibility, relatedness in outcomes, dose-response relationship, etc.). We also review the exclusions. Exclusion of patients otherwise likely to experience side-effects may affect generalizability of results of adverse events reporting (e.g., it may happen if patients are restricted to those who are not naïve to an intervention or may occur through a run-in and exclusion period). We review drop-outs due to adverse effects. If composite endpoints are used for efficacy, we note whether they are used for safety. We take a conservative approach to adverse events for new agents. We also remain aware that there is a potential for overreacting to possible harms reported in low quality studies, which, again, can ultimately be harmful to patients in other ways if no reasonable alternatives are available.

~~~

Evaluating Authors' Conclusions

The first important point to make is that authors' conclusions are generally opinions, even when they're making strong sounding claims. And we remind you again that it may be helpful to assume a certain amount of bias or "rooting for the study intervention" on the part of the researchers, even if wholly innocently and unconsciously. One helpful tip is to always be mindful that not all associations are causal, and often associations should be examined in the reverse.

Reversal of Direction, Reversal of Fortune

A good example comes from our Vioxx case study in which the authors stated, "[Our] results are consistent with the theory that naproxen has a coronary protective effect and highlight the fact that rofecoxib does not provide this type of protection owing to its selective inhibition of cyclooxygenase-2 at its therapeutic doses and at higher doses." Readers applying critical thinking would look at statements such as this and come up with alternate possibilities. (*Oh, like the opposite could be true!*)

More Reversals: Confounding by Indication

This brings us to another example, which also highlights the great potential for misleading outcomes in observational studies and some clinical trials. Confounding-by-indication is a bias that occurs when unblinded clinicians tailor interventions to meet the needs of specific patients, frequently creating a selection bias. For example, if a new antidepressant is known—or believed—to decrease the risk of suicide, many doctors will put their highest risk patients on the new antidepressant, leaving stable patients on older antidepressants. When investigators examine their databases, they see that the suicide rate is higher in the patients who took the new antidepressant. Why? The answer is that the database study was biased by "confounding by indication."

Confounding by indication is common in clinical practice and observational studies because clinicians prescribe different drugs for patients with different demographic or clinical characteristics such as age, condition, severity of illness or comorbid conditions in order to achieve best results for individual patients. Effective randomization and successful blinding (which includes successful concealment of allocation) prevents confounding by indication.

When You Hear Research Results

So keep in mind, when hearing about cause-and-effect claims, determine if the study is an experiment or an observation. If it is an observation, be wary unless the results are "all-or-none," which, again, are very, very rare. If it is an experiment, is it valid? And remember that some claims invite asking a question, "What came first? Chicken or egg? Was this spun one way? Should the spin be reversed?" In short, which is the cause and which is the effect?

~~~

Evidence Grading

Evidence grading is simply a tag of a summary conclusion about the quality of a study or other item or element such as a body of evidence, a clinical guideline or a clinical recommendation, for example. At times, we rate the "body of evidence" and refer to it as the overall "strength of evidence" (SOE).

Whenever you see an evidence grade, it is vitally important that you make sure you understand the criteria for achieving a specific grade. Many grading systems may use similar words, but have very different criteria. And unfortunately, many criteria upgrade trials so that trials may be given a high grade when in fact they are not valid.

When we are performing systematic reviews, we often utilize our modification of the system used by the AHRQ-EHCP (the Agency for Healthcare Research and Quality and the Effective Health Care Program). But for practical and teaching purposes, we have a very simple system, the criteria for which essentially are your judgment about the distorting effects of bias and chance and your assessment of clinical significance.

The Delfini grading system is designed to be easy to understand, easy to remember and flexible to apply. The concepts behind our grading system can be applied to individual studies or outcomes or conclusions from studies, systematic reviews, clinical recommendations, guidelines, etc. Most frequently, we grade studies, outcomes and SOE using a system of A, B, B-U or U. At times we rate the SOE as high, moderate, borderline or inconclusive. We use A, B and B-U to inform efficacy decisions. Grade U evidence is rarely used by us to inform efficacy decisions, but may be used for safety, but with cautionary statements that the evidence is of uncertain reliability.

Grade A: Useful

The evidence is strong and appears sufficient to use in making health care decisions—it is both valid and useful (e.g., meets standards for clinical significance, sufficient magnitude of effect size, physician and patient acceptability, etc.). Studies achieving this grade should be outstanding in design, methodology, execution and reporting and have successful study performance outcomes, providing useful information to aid clinical decision-making, enabling reasonable certitude in drawing conclusions.

For a body of evidence: Several well-designed and conducted studies that consistently show similar results.

For therapy, screening and prevention: RCTs. In some cases a single, large Grade A RCT may be sufficient; however, without confirmation from other studies, results could be due to chance, undetected significant biases, fraud, etc. In such instance, the SOE should include a cautionary note.

Grade A should be rarely assigned to any study. ("Extra points" are not given for challenge or difficulty in answering the research question. Authors should not be given extra points by second-guessing them. Transparency is required.)

Grade B: Possibly Useful

Grade B studies should be very well designed and executed and meet most of the requirements that it takes to achieve a Grade A. Grade B evidence appears potentially strong and is probably sufficient to use in making health care decisions—some threats to validity have been identified. Studies achieving this grade should be of high quality and contain only non-lethal threats to validity and with sufficiently useful information to aid clinical decision-making, enabling reasonable certitude in drawing conclusions.

For a body of evidence: The evidence is strong enough to conclude that the results are probably valid and useful (see above); however, study results from multiple studies are inconsistent or the studies may have some (but not lethal) threats to validity.

For therapy, screening and prevention: RCTs. In some cases a single, large Grade B RCT may be sufficient; however, without confirmation from other studies results could be due to chance, undetected significant biases, fraud, etc. In such instance, the SOE should include a cautionary note.

Grade B is more frequent than Grade A, but is still a difficult grade to achieve.

Grade B-U: Possible to Uncertain Usefulness

The evidence might be sufficient to use in making health care decisions; however, there remains sufficient uncertainty that the evidence cannot fully reach a Grade B, and the uncertainty is not great enough to fully warrant a Grade U.

Grade U: Uncertain Validity and/or Usefulness

There is sufficient uncertainty that caution is urged regarding its use in making health care decisions. Grade U should be assigned when there is sufficient uncertainty about the accuracy of the estimates of effect resulting in an inability to comfortably draw conclusions from the research and in comfortably applying results.

We end up assigning most studies a Grade U. As stated, we generally never use Grade U studies to inform efficacy decisions, but we will use Grade U evidence for safety, being very careful to describe that the evidence is of low quality.

For readers who would like more detailed information about other systems, a good place to start is a publication from the Agency for Healthcare and Research and Quality and the online Cochrane Handbook [Owens, Higgins]. We also have additional information available at our website.

Tips and Tools

One bottom line is that we like to see several valid studies done in slightly different ways by groups with different interests (diluting potential conflicts) with consistent results to feel we have arrived at "truth!"

A very big bottom line is USE TOOLS! Find critical appraisal tools that you like and which will not lead you into trouble. For example, avoid relying upon JADAD scoring at all cost! (It is a highly inadequate method even though it is frequently used by systematic reviewers.) We invite you to use our freely available tools at the Delfini Library. The important point is to find critical appraisal tools that you like and that are likely to lead you to a valid assessment of a study.

We emphasize use of tools because they help remind you of what to assess and help remind you of what is a threat to validity because of what is missing.

How We Read A Study

A joke that we frequently tell our workshop participants is that we don't really "read" studies. After taking a quick look as described above in **Quick Tips for Initially Assessing Possible Usefulness of a Clinical Trial**, we peruse the study hunting for any critical appraisal element that we will want to make note of. Sheri does this by hand by writing small abbreviations of each study element of interest in the margin. Mike does this online. Any mention relating to blinding, for example, may be coded as BLD. This method makes it very easy to find anything having to do with blinding so that blinding can be considered all at once after this coding step has been completed. Other notes or notations, such as minus signs to represent problem areas, may be added to the margins. We then take our short critical appraisal checklist and quickly scan it for anything that might not have been mentioned in the study.

This coding process takes only a few minutes, and frequently this may be all that we need to determine study quality. Another advantage of this method is that it results in instant documentation, plus it makes it very easy to engage in study discussions because it is very easy to find key study information.

If we have to do a formal write-up, we have found it very expedient to simply copy the abstract out of PubMed into a Word document, add any key elements missing from the abstract (it is very rare that we have to do this), and then list our threats to validity underneath followed by our grade, a grading tag and a concluding statement.

Other Study Issues

As we explained in the outset, our primary focus for this book is on **evaluating the reliability and clinical usefulness** of **efficacy results** of **superiority trials** of **therapeutic interventions.** In this section, we will give you **a few tips** for areas for which you may need some additional information, help for which is freely available at our website.

Again, **this is not comprehensive**—but just to give you some **warnings and pointers** for other special study areas. A deeper dive, as you need it, is recommended. We have resources freely available on our website for the issues touched upon below. These areas are—

- Oncology Study Outcomes

- Comparative Study Designs: Equivalence and Non-inferiority Studies

- Cross-over Designs

- Studies of Diagnostic Testing

- Studies of Screening Tests

- Reminders about Secondary Studies and Secondary Sources

Oncology Study Outcomes

A key problem with oncology studies centers around study outcomes. Endpoint quality can be ranked as follows:

1. Death

2. Death plus tumor assessment judgments

3. Tumor assessment judgments

Some key points include the following. In addition to usual biases in clinical trials, there is a higher likelihood of bias and the risk of potentially misleading results when studies are small and brief and when survival is not the primary outcome measure.

Progression-free survival (PFS) may be a composite endpoint including tumor response. Tumor response may not be a good proxy for survival even if assessment is blinded. Tumor measurements may mislead because they may not correlate with full tumor burden, mortality and other outcomes of importance to patients. Toxicity of treatment may be so great that patients die from it even if a tumor is stable or shrinking.

Quality of life and functioning may be important endpoints to study in absence of true survival information. Overall survival differences, even when statistically significant, may be small.

A table of typical oncology outcomes and key considerations is available on our website.

Comparative Study Designs: Equivalence and Non-inferiority Trials

This is a complex area, and we recommend downloading our freely available 1-page summary to help assess these other comparative study designs. Here is a short sampling of some of the problems in these designs: lack of sufficient evidence confirming efficacy of referent treatment, ("referent" refers to the comparator treatment); study not sufficiently similar to referent study; inappropriate Deltas (meaning the margin established for equivalence or non-inferiority); or significant biases or analysis methods that would tend to diminish an effect size and "favor" no difference between groups (e.g., conservative application of ITT analysis, insufficient power, etc.), thus pushing toward non-inferiority or equivalence.

Cross-over Designs

This too is a complex area, and we recommend downloading our freely available 1-page summary to help you assess these trials. There are special problems that result when a subject is serving as his or her own control, and these designs must be evaluated carefully. For example, sequencing treatments must be randomized, blinding must be handled carefully and may be at a greater risk of failure, potential for carry-over effects must be guarded against, loss of data is magnified and calculations may be at greater risk of error due to complexity.

Studies of Diagnostic Tests

Having just described a couple of other study areas as complex, evaluating studies of diagnostic tests is even *more* complex. For information on this topic, we recommend that you download our full **Study Validity and Usability Tool** freely available at our website.

Here are some of the key requirements for evaluating diagnostic studies, in shorthand. The new test requires better outcomes or value. The test should be compared to a gold standard or a reasonable comparator and find the same abnormality and within the same time period that does not result in a change in diagnosis. The test should be applied to all or a random sample of subjects with and without disease. Assessors should be blinded. There should be minimal bias from indeterminate results. Measures of test function need to be clinically useful.

Studies of Screening Tests

Screening is a hot and frequently emotional topic. When it comes to screening, there are some special bias considerations. For information on this topic, we recommend that you download our full **Study Validity and Usability Tool** freely available at our website.

Here are some of the key requirements, in shorthand. Early diagnosis and treatments determined to be effective should improve outcomes more than later diagnosis and treatment. Beneficial outcomes should be examined for risk of the operation of some special biases that are uniquely problematic in screening tests (e.g., lead time bias, length bias, overdiagnosis or volunteer bias are some special biases that can plague studies of screening tests).

Secondary Studies and Secondary Sources

As we stated at the start of this book, by a secondary study, we mean a study of studies such as a systematic review, an example of which would be a meta-analysis. By a secondary source, we mean any information source that utilizes primary and secondary studies. Examples include health care economic studies, clinical practice guidelines, compendia, decision support, etc.

At this point, it should come as no surprise to you that many secondary studies and secondary sources cannot be relied upon. This is largely because many primary studies are not reliable and because frequently an effective critical appraisal is not performed. But then the primary studies are used in the secondary studies and sources anyway.

At this point, it should also come as no surprise to you that we have help freely available on our website in the form of tools that you can download to critically appraise secondary studies and secondary sources.

~~~

Summary

Health care decisions we make and actions we take should be based on reliable evidence when it exists. Determining if health care evidence is reliable requires critical appraisal for validity and clinical usefulness. In this book, we have focused on how we assess medical research dealing with therapeutic interventions. Our approach relies on a basic understanding of bias, confounding and chance and how to assess studies to determine if there is a likely cause and effect association between the therapy and important outcomes. If we can rule out bias, confounding and chance through critical appraisal, and the benefits are clinically meaningful with acceptable risks, patient should be made aware of the results and the quality of the evidence as part of health care decision-making.

Our approach is to examine and assess the risk of bias in the 4 areas of a clinical trial and look for any potential biases or differences in—

- Demographic or clinical variables in study groups;

- Interventions, care experiences or other contextual elements of the study; and,

- Data acquisition and management or assessments of outcomes in the study groups which might distort the reported study efficacy or safety results.

We also look for other threats to validity which will vary from study to study, e.g., other biases, selective reporting of results, etc.

We always use a tool.

We grade evidence using a simple but useful system of A, B, B-U and U.

We hope that the information provided in this book will make it possible for readers to more effectively and efficiently evaluate clinical trials and other medical evidence.

READER RESOURCE WEB PAGE

For tools and online resources:

http://www.delfinigrouppublishing.com/ResourcesEvaluatingClinicalTrials.htm

~~~

ABOUT THE AUTHORS

Delfini Group is a public service entrepreneurship founded to advance applied evidence- and value-based clinical quality improvements and methods through practice, training and facilitation. Much of Delfini's work is dedicated to help solve the little known societal problem of medical misinformation. Delfini has contributed to text books, advised government entities, worked with health care systems, payers and manufacturers and has trained thousands of health care professionals in evidence-based quality improvement.

Michael E. Stuart MD & Sheri Ann Strite are medical information scientists, medical evidologists and evidence-based clinical improvement experts who combine academic and practical experience to—

- Train people how to evaluate medical research studies.

- Conduct evidence reviews.

- Help health care systems apply evidence- and value-based clinical quality improvement methods including special help for work groups such as clinical guideline development teams, pharmacy & therapeutics and medical technology assessment committees, clinical quality improvement teams, journal clubs and more.

- Train physicians and others in communicating with patients.

Sheri Ann Strite, Co-founder, Principal & Managing Partner, initiated many Delfini health care improvement strategies, tools and training programs including the popular Delfini critical appraisal training program. Formerly she was Associate Director, Program Development, University of California, San Diego (UCSD) Family & Preventive Medicine, School of Medicine, where she taught faculty, physicians, residents, medical and pharmacy students and medical librarians. She was also a member of the UCSD Family Medicine Research Leaders and faculty for their Research Fellowship in the Department of Family & Preventive Medicine. Prior to UCSD, Ms. Strite worked in clinical improvement, education and research at Group Health Cooperative in Seattle, Washington, where she held various positions including leadership and research management and administration.

Michael E. Stuart MD, Co-founder, President & Medical Director, is a family physician and was appointed a clinical faculty position at the University of Washington in 1975. He is the former Director of the Department of Clinical Improvement and Education at Group Health Cooperative in Seattle, Washington, where he led development of more than 35 evidence-based clinical guidelines and other clinical improvements, chaired the Pharmacy & Therapeutics and Medical Technology Assessment Committees. His work has received praise from prominent health care leaders such as David Eddy MD, Don Berwick MD, Health Ministry of New Zealand and the US Navy Bureau of Medicine.

Topics upon which Delfini has written and taught include critical appraisal of medical literature, evidence-based committee processes, health care content development, technology assessment, population-based care, projecting economic and health outcomes, performance measurement, patient decision-making, facilitating provider behavior change, physician/patient communications, developing and implementing clinical guidelines, and creating information, decision and action aids for clinical care.

~~~

THANKS

We hope that this little book, which represents years of our hard labor, will result in smoothing your way to understanding how to evaluate a clinical trial. We would appreciate your review at Amazon or other publication outlets. And you can contact us via our website at http://www.delfini.org.

~~~

REFERENCES

Atkins D, Chang S, Gartlehner G, Buckley DI, Whitlock EP, Berliner E, Matchar D. Assessing the Applicability of Studies When Comparing Medical Interventions. 2010 Dec 30. Methods Guide for Effectiveness and Comparative Effectiveness Reviews [Internet]. Rockville (MD): Agency for Health care Research and Quality (US); 2008-. Available from http://www.ncbi.nlm.nih.gov/books/NBK53480/ PubMed PMID: 21433409.

Bombardier C, Laine L, Reicin A, Shapiro D, Burgos-Vargas R, Davis B, Day R, Ferraz MB, Hawkey CJ, Hochberg MC, Kvien TK, Schnitzer TJ; VIGOR Study Group. Comparison of upper gastrointestinal toxicity of rofecoxib and naproxen in patients with rheumatoid arthritis. VIGOR Study Group. N Engl J Med. 2000 Nov 23;343(21):1520-8, 2 p following 1528. PubMed PMID: 11087881.

Carpenter J.R, Kenward M.G. Missing data in randomized controlled trials—a practical guide http://www.hta.nhs.uk/nihrmethodology/reports/1589.pdf.

Chalmers TC, Celano P, Sacks HS, Smith H Jr. Bias in treatment assignment in controlled clinical trials. N Engl J Med. 1983 Dec 1;309(22):1358-61. PubMed PMID: 6633598.

Consumer Affairs at http://www.consumeraffairs.com/news04/vioxx_estimates.html#ixzz0cqOwLu3m

COTS: Canadian Orthopaedic Trauma Society. Nonoperative treatment compared with plate fixation of displaced midshaft clavicular fractures. A multicenter, randomized clinical trial. J Bone Joint Surg Am. 2007 Jan;89(1):1-10. PubMed PMID: 17200303.

Digital History at http://www.digitalhistory.uh.edu/era.cfm?eraid=18&smtid=1

Echt DS, Liebson PR, Mitchell LB, et al. Mortality and morbidity in patients receiving encainide, flecainide, or placebo. The Cardiac Arrhythmia Suppression Trial. N Engl J Med. 1991 Mar 21;324(12):781-8. PubMed PMID: 1900101.

Field MJ, Lohr KN, eds. Guidelines for Clinical Practice: From Development to Use. Washington, DC: National Academies Press; 1992.

Freedman, David H. Lies, Damn Lies and Bad Medical Science. The Atlantic. November, 2010. www.theatlantic.com/magazine/archive/2010/11/lies-damned-lies-and-medical-science/8269/, accessed 11/07/2010.

Glasziou P. The EBM journal selection process: how to find the 1 in 400 valid and highly relevant new research articles. Evid Based Med. 2006 Aug;11(4):101. PubMed PMID: 17213115.

Gotzsche PC. Believability of relative risks and odds ratios in abstracts: cross sectional study. BMJ 2006;333;231-234; PMID: 16854948.

Hartling L, Ospina M, Liang Y, Dryden DM, Hooton N, Krebs Seida J, Klassen TP. Risk of bias versus quality assessment of randomised controlled trials: cross sectional study. BMJ. 2009 Oct 19;339:b4012. doi: 10.1136/bmj.b4012. PubMed PMID: 19841007; PubMed Central PMCID: PMC2764034.

Higgins JPT, Green S (editors). Cochrane Handbook for Systematic Reviews of Interventions Version 5.1.0 [updated March 2011]. The Cochrane Collaboration, 2011. Available from www.cochrane-handbook.org. Section 8.2.1. Accessed 11/9/12.

Ioannidis JP, Haidich AB, Lau J. Any casualties in the clash of randomised and observational evidence? BMJ. 2001 Apr 14;322(7291):879-80.PMID: 11302887

Ioannidis JPA. Why Most Published Research Findings are False. PLoS Med 2005; 2(8):696 701. PMID: 16060722

Julius S, Nesbitt SD, Egan BM, et al. Trial of Preventing Hypertension (TROPHY) Study Investigators. Feasibility of treating prehypertension with an angiotensin-receptor blocker. N Engl J Med. 2006 Apr 20;354(16):1685-97. Epub 2006 Mar 14. PubMed PMID: 16537662.

Juni P, Altman DG, Egger M (2001) Systematic reviews in health care: assessing the quality of controlled clinical trials. BMJ 2001;323:42-6.PubMed PMID: 11440947

Juni P, Witschi A, Bloch R, Egger M. The hazards of scoring the quality of clinical trials for meta-analysis. JAMA. 1999 Sep 15;282(11):1054-60. PubMed PMID: 10493204.

Kaptchuk TJ, Kelley JM, Conboy LA, et al. Components of placebo effect: randomised controlled trial in patients with irritable bowel syndrome. BMJ. 2008 May 3;336(7651):999-1003. Epub 2008 Apr 3. PubMed PMID: 18390493.

Kjaergard LL, Villumsen J, Gluud C. Reported methodological quality and discrepancies between large and small randomized trials in metaanalyses. Ann Intern Med 2001;135:982–89. PMID 11730399

Lachin JM (filed as Lachin JL). Statistical considerations in the intent-to-treat principle. Control Clin Trials. 2000 Oct;21(5):526. PubMed PMID: 11018568. Erratum: Refers to John M. Lachin: http://www.sciencedirect.com/science/article/pii/S0197245600000921

Marciniak TA. Memorandum of June 14, 2010 on cardiovascular events in RECORD (NDA 21-071/S-035): FDA briefing document, pages 16-151. http://www.fda.gov/AdvisoryCommittees/Calendar/ucm214612.htm. Accessed July 9, 2010.

McKibbon KA, Wilczynski NL, Haynes RB. What do evidence-based secondary journals tell us about the publication of clinically important articles in primary health care journals? BMC Med. 2004 Sep 6;2:33. Pubmed PMID: 15350200

Merck Newsroom:
http://bus8010lewis.alliant.wikispaces.net/file/view/Merck+Newsroom+Executive+Speech es.txt accessed 10/23/2012

Moher D, Pham B, Jones A, Cook DJ, Jadad AR, Moher M, Tugwell P, Klassen TP. Does quality of reports of randomised trials affect estimates of intervention efficacy reported in meta-analyses? Lancet. 1998 Aug 22;352(9128):609-13. PubMed PMID: 9746022.

Morganroth J, Bigger JT Jr, Anderson JL. Treatment of ventricular arrhythmias by United States cardiologists: a survey before the Cardiac Arrhythmia Suppression Trial results were available. Am J Cardiol. 1990 Jan 1;65(1):40-8. PubMed PMID: 1688481.

Mundell EJ and Gardner A. Journal Corrects Vioxx Article to Reflect Short-Term Heart Risk. 2006. http://news.healingwell.com/index.php?p=news1&id=533482. Accessed 5/31/2013.

Nissen SE, Wolski K. Effect of rosiglitazone on the risk of myocardial infarction and death from cardiovascular causes. N Engl J Med. 2007 Jun 14;356(24):2457-71. Epub 2007 May 21. Erratum in: N Engl J Med. 2007 Jul 5;357(1):100.. PubMed PMID: 17517853.

Nuesch E, Trelle S, Reichenbach S, Rutjes AW, Bürgi E, et al. (2009) The effects of excluding patients from the analysis in randomized controlled trials: meta-epidemiological study. BMJ 339:b3244. doi: 10.1136. PMID: 19736281

O'Brien PC, Zhang D, Bailey KR. Semi-parametric and non-parametric methods for clinical trials with incomplete data. Stat Med. 2005 Feb 15;24(3):341-58. Erratum in: Stat Med. 2005 Nov 15;24(21):3385. PMID: 15547952

Owens DK, Lohr KN, Atkins D, et al.AHRQ series paper 5: grading the strength of a body of evidence when comparing medical interventions--agency for health care research and quality and the effective health-care program. J Clin Epidemiol. 2010 May;63(5):513-23. PubMed PMID: 19595577.

Patel A. ADVANCE Collaborative Group, MacMahon S, et al. Effects of a fixed combination of perindopril and indapamide on macrovascular and microvascular outcomes in patients with type 2 diabetes mellitus (the ADVANCE trial): a randomised controlled trial. Lancet. 2007 Sep 8;370(9590):829-40.PubMed PMID: 17765963.

Pitkin RM, Branagan MA, Burmeister LF. Accuracy of data in abstracts of published research articles. JAMA. 1999 Mar 24-31;281(12):1110-1. PubMed PMID:10188662.

Poolman RW, Struijs PA, Krips R, Inger N. Sierevelt IN, et al. (2007) Reporting of outcomes in orthopaedic randomized trials: Does blinding of outcome assessors matter? J Bone Joint Surg Am. 89:550–558. PMID 17332104

Psaty BM, Prentice RL. Minimizing bias in randomized trials: the importance of blinding. JAMA. 2010 Aug 18;304(7):793-4. PubMed PMID: 20716744.

Reichenbach S, Sterchi R, Scherer M, et al. Meta-analysis: chondroitin for osteoarthritis of the knee or hip. Ann Intern Med. 2007 Apr 17;146(8):580-90. PubMed PMID: 17438317.

Savovic J, Jones HE, Altman DG, et al. Influence of Reported Study Design Characteristics on Intervention Effect Estimates From Randomized, Controlled Trials. Ann Intern Med. 2012 Sep 4. doi: 10.7326/0003-4819-157-6-201209180-00537. [Epub ahead of print] PubMed PMID: 22945832.

Schulz KF, Chalmers I, Hayes RJ, Altman D. Empirical evidence of bias. Dimensions of methodological quality associated with estimates of treatment effects in controlled trials. JAMA 1995;273:408–12. PMID: 7823387

Shih W. Problems in dealing with missing data and informative censoring in clinical trials. Curr Control Trials Cardiovasc Med. 2002 Jan 8;3(1):4. PubMed PMID: 11985778; PubMed Central PMCID: PMC134476.

Tierney JF, Stewart LA. Investigating patient exclusion bias in meta-analysis. Int J Epidemiol. 2005 Feb;34(1):79-87. Epub 2004 Nov 23. PubMed PMID: 15561753.

van Tulder MW, Suttorp M, Morton S, et al. Empirical evidence of an association between internal validity and effect size in randomized controlled trials of low-back pain. Spine (Phila Pa 1976). 2009 Jul 15;34(16):1685-92. PubMed PMID: 19770609.

Made in the USA
Lexington, KY
29 July 2013